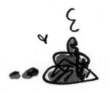

THE LIFE OF
POO

To Donna – thank you. For everything.

ADAM HART

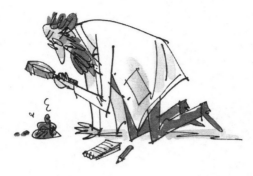

THE LIFE OF
POO

*or why you should think
twice about shaking hands
(especially with men)*

KYLE BOOKS

First published in Great Britain in 2015 by
Kyle Books, an imprint of Kyle Cathie Ltd.
192–198 Vauxhall Bridge Road
London SW1V 1DX
general.enquiries@kylebooks.com
www.kylebooks.com

10 9 8 7 6 5 4 3 2 1

ISBN 978 0 85783 292 4

Editor: Judith Hannam
Designer: Peter Ward
Illustrator: Marie-Hélène Jeeves
Production: Lisa Pinnell

A Cataloguing in Publication record for this title is available
from the British Library.

Printed and bound by CPI Group (UK) Ltd, Croydon, CR0 4YY

Contents

CHAPTER ONE

Are You Sitting Comfortably?

We begin this journey by sitting on the toilet. For the sake of maintaining some dignity you can *imagine* you are sitting on the toilet, although a study by the Imperial Cancer Fund in 2001 suggests that around 40% of readers may not need to resort to imagination. This study, which relied on people's honesty in a personal matter, so almost certainly underestimated the true occurrence, found that 49% of men and 26% of women confuse the bathroom with a library.[1] Sadly, data does not exist for the opposite confusion.

I'd like you to imagine that you have just done a poo, laid a cable, released the little brown fish, composted the worms or whatever euphemism you prefer for the act of defecation. Alternatively, if you are reading this on the toilet and are engaged in a 'gardening project', then take a quick peek between your legs (don't pretend you've never done it) at the poo you have produced.

Let's assume that you are healthy and your bowel is in good shape. You eat a balanced diet with the right amount of fibre and other components that make for 'good stool'. Delicious, lovingly prepared food has gone in one end, beautiful in colour and texture, and yet it has emerged the other end as a badly smelling, uniformly brown, uniformly textured, slightly spongy (take my word for it) cracked cylinder. Clearly something profound has occurred in your gut.

It is tempting to think of the gut, or more technically the gastrointestinal tract, as a simple tube that goes from the mouth to the anus, slowly converting nice food to nasty poo. A sort of fleshy sewerage system that extracts what we need from our food and then expels what we don't, sometimes propelled by a gaseous by-product of the process. However, this view of the gut is extremely simplistic. It is like looking at a rainforest and reducing all of our understanding and knowledge of its incredible complexity of function and biodiversity to the simple fact that it's very green and rather damp.

Take a look at that poo again. Does it look like undigested food? Clearly it doesn't – it is far too uniform in colour and texture. Does it smell like undigested food? If it does, then you really need to look at what you are eating. Poo doesn't smell anything like food, even food that has been chewed up and left for a couple of days.

Analysis of poo reveals that, like many things biological, it is mostly (75%) water. Of the remaining appropriately termed solid fraction, some is cholesterol and other fatty substances, there's a little protein in there, and some inorganic compounds like the calcium phosphate that makes up a high proportion of bones and teeth enamel. There's some indigestible food, like cellulose and components of dietary fibre (which we'll touch on in Chapter Eight and discuss in more depth in Chapter Ten) and you can also find, if you look under a microscope, cells from the wall of the gut. These are shed as poo passes down through the intestine and into the rectum, which is the foyer to the anus's back door. (It's these cells that allow forensic scientists to gather DNA from faeces that are, for some reason, commonly left behind by burglars during break-ins.)

If you turn up the magnification on your microscope, you'll also see that about a third of the solid material, and sometimes up to 60%, is bacteria. It is the bacteria that are responsible both for mass and for smell. It is also the presence of millions of these single-celled organisms in our poo that gives us a big clue about what's actually going on in our gut.

Introducing bacteria

Bacteria are living organisms that reproduce, move about and consume resources (gases from the air and food from the environment around them) just like we do. However, there are some significant differences in the way they go about their lives, as we'll see later. For now, though, there are three very important facts that are worth bearing in mind about bacteria.

They are very small

Bacteria are single-celled organisms, so you're not expecting them to be big, but many cells, including human egg cells, some cells that make up the nervous systems and the pond-dwelling amoeba from

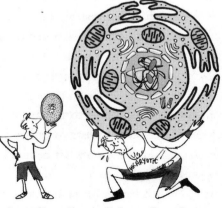

Prokaryotic cell   Eukaryotic cell

biology lessons, are actually visible to the naked eye. Many of the rest don't need more than a simple microscope to see them. Bacteria are very much smaller than these cells, partly because, unlike the cells we usually think about, bacterial cells lack a nucleus (the large structure that contains DNA) and most other internal structures. They are known as prokaryotes, and their cells are *prokaryotic* (lacking a nucleus). They do have DNA, but it is in the form of a single circular chromosome. This simplicity of structure allows them to be very tiny, typically 10–100 times smaller in diameter than the so-called *eukaryotic cells* (cells with a nucleus) that make up our bodies and the bodies of all the plants, animals and fungi on Earth.

They are very numerous

A millilitre of water, which is barely more than an enthusiastic drop, might contain a million bacteria, and a gram of soil (you probably have more lurking in the tread of your shoe) can contain 40 million. Their small size and ability to live almost anywhere lead to a global population with a biomass exceeding that of all the plants and animals combined. It is estimated that there are approximately 5×10^{30} bacteria on Earth, or 5,000,000,000,000, 000,000,000,000,000,000, which is a very big number any way you want to look at it.[2] All the seconds that have ticked by since the Big Bang don't even come close.

They are very good at what they do

It's an understatement to say that bacteria are extraordinarily good at what they do. They are staggeringly effective at exploiting all that Earth has to offer. They live on, in and around almost anywhere and anything. Whether you are looking at the bottom of the ocean, in the rock underneath the bottom of the ocean, high in the atmosphere, deep in the Earth's crust, in hot springs,

Just how big is 5×10^{30}, or 5,000,000,000,000,000,000,000,000,000,000?

The Big Bang that started the universe was 14,000,000,000 years ago.

Every second since the Big Bang

= 14,000,000,000 x 365 (days)
  x 24 (hours) x 60 (minutes) x 60 (seconds)
= 441,504,000,000,000,000 seconds

This huge number is more than 11 *billion times smaller* than the number of bacteria on Earth!

How about this:

The Earth weighs about 6×10^{24} kg (6,000,000,000,000, 000,000,000,000 kg).

There are about 50 grains of rice to a gram, so if each bacterium weighed as much as a grain of rice, they would collectively weigh 16.7 *times more* than the Earth! This also demonstrates just how very tiny bacteria are.

deep underneath polar ice, on the surface of your eyeball, on your food, in your dog's saliva, in an earwig's ear, up a flea's backside or in your gut, you'll find them. Bacteria can live almost everywhere and their unique biology, their ubiquity and their sheer weight of numbers make them more than just a force to be reckoned with. Their activities shape and define much of the world around us as well as the world within us.

Exploring how some of these bacterial activities affect our

lives is what this book is all about, and an easy place to start our exploration is where food starts its transformation into poo: the mouth.

Open wide!

You probably think of your mouth as a convenient place to shove food and to do some chewing before swallowing. As a functional description of the mouth, 'food hole' does a reasonable job, but to understand the role bacteria have in our lives we need to start thinking of our bodies ecologically as a human ecosystem.

Ecologically, the human mouth is a tremendously complex network of habitats. Teeth, gums, lips, tongue and palate all present different opportunities for bacteria that are able to colonise them, and the warm and wet conditions are ideal for their growth. In fact, more than 750 different types of bacteria have been identified from the oral cavity and, depending on how you define 'type' (something that can be difficult with bacteria), some studies estimate that the total number might reach 25,000.[3] In other words, no matter how scrupulous your oral hygiene, right now your mouth is awash with abundant and diverse bacteria.

Studying bacteria in the mouth, or indeed anywhere, used to rely solely on our ability to culture them. In bacterial culturing, Petri dishes are filled with growth medium, generally a gel-like substance containing specific nutrients required for the target bacterial types to grow. The bacteria are transferred from the place of interest to the surface of that medium by a swab, a water droplet or some other means. They then grow on what is called the 'plate' until they are present in sufficient numbers to form bacterial colonies, generally visible to the naked eye. These colonies provide the cells for whatever studies we might want to undertake. The problem is that most bacteria simply won't grow on plates; we can't culture them. In fact, those we can culture are only a small fraction of the diversity that is out there, even though we are developing techniques to improve our culturing success all the time.[4]

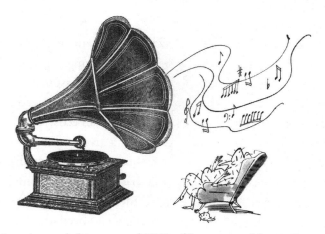

It's estimated that around 50% of human oral bacteria cannot be cultured, although analysis of their genetic material (their DNA) tells us they are there. Our understanding of their role, and the development of that understanding over recent years, provides a useful lesson in how we should be considering bacteria in general.

Why we should be grateful to the son of a Dutch basket maker

Oral bacteria were first described, and this is hard to believe if you're not 'up' on early microscopy, in the mid-seventeenth century. Nearly 350 years ago, using a tiny ball of glass as a lens, Antony van Leeuwenhoek, the son of a Dutch basket maker, described bacteria

we now know as *selenomonads* that he
gathered from the inside of, presumably,
his own mouth. His microscope didn't look
anything like a modern
microscope and was
incredibly fiddly to
use, but nonetheless
his descriptions of
oral bacteria weren't
improved on that
much even with
the development of
electron microscopes.

Microbiology (as the
study of bacteria became known) progressed and oral bacteria were
among the first that we learned to culture. However, despite all this
progress, it took until the 1960s for us to prove the link between
oral bacteria living on our teeth (a bacterium called *Streptococcus
mutans*) and tooth decay, and until the 1980s for the link between
bacteria and periodontal (gum) disease to be widely recognised.

My point here is two-fold. The first point is that despite our
having discovered them early, their being relatively easy to culture
(at least, a few of them) and our being interested in studying them,
it took a fair while for the importance of oral bacteria in human
health to be appreciated. Clearly, proving bacterial links to disease
can be a difficult business. The second point is more subtle, but
potentially more important. Initial studies of bacterial interactions
with our oral cavity were disease-centred. We asked the question
how does this bacterium (singular) make us ill? What we are now
starting to realise is that we should be asking how do these bacteria
(plural) make us ill *and* how do they keep us well? Increasingly,

those are the questions we are asking of bacteria throughout the human ecosystem.

Bacterial communities and microbe micro-cities

If we were dealing with animals and plants in a particular habitat, then we would refer to the collection of different types (or different *species*) that were present as a *community*. We can apply exactly the same ecological language to the collection of bacteria present in our mouths, or anywhere else in the rich range of habitats we provide for them. Thus, we have the oral community, the intestinal community and the rectal community, all of whom probably feel superior to the anal community. Another term used to describe these communities of bacteria is *flora*. Technically, flora means the flower species that grow in a particular area, but the word has been borrowed by microbiology and it is common to hear reference to 'gut flora'. *Microbiota* (literally 'small life') is perhaps a better term and can refer to bacteria as well as to other microbes, such as yeasts, which are fungi. An uncomfortable mix of the two, *microflora* is another term sometimes used.

Whatever we call them, we are increasingly interested in these communities, in groups of interacting bacteria, rather than focusing on a single bacterial type and its potential for harm. Tooth decay is a case in point. We know now that decayed regions of a tooth have a far more complex array of bacteria types than just *Streptomyces mutans*. Seventy-five different types of bacteria have been identified from decayed teeth and 31 have been identified in a single decay lesion.[5] Similarly, hundreds of different bacterial types have been identified in areas of gum disease.

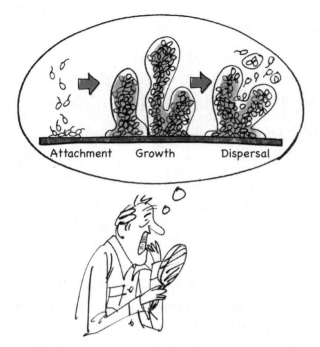

Attachment   Growth   Dispersal

It is a tremendously complex world in our mouths, and bacteria, just like other organisms, have a complex set of interactions with one another. Bacteria exist on surfaces like our teeth and tongue as a biofilm, which we can actually feel on the surface of our teeth, assuming we haven't very recently brushed them. A bacterial biofilm is an assemblage of different bacterial species embedded within what is called the extracellular polymeric substance (EPS). The EPS is secreted by the cells themselves and can have a distinct three-dimensional architecture. That sticky layer on your teeth is a bacterial city of multiple, interacting, bacterial species that you callously destroy every time you brush.

Bacteria = bad?

The crucial thing with bacterial communities, just as with cities, is that not everyone dwelling within them is bad, no matter how seductive the 'bacteria = bad' equation might be. I just checked my thesaurus and the suggested alternative for bacteria is 'germ', which is hardly a positive synonym. It's not surprising that this is the case, because bacteria certainly do cause diseases: anthrax, botulism, cholera, diphtheria, Lyme disease, salmonella, scarlet fever, syphilis, tetanus, tooth decay (which seems rather trivial in this list), tuberculosis . . . oh, and bubonic plague, to name but a few of the better known. But they're far from being all bad.

It's all about balance

A city may have some muggers and murderers, but most people are pretty decent and their positive actions tend to vastly outweigh the negative actions of the harmful minority. There's a balance in a well-established community that helps to make that community stable. In principle, the oral bacterial community is no different: processes like competing for limited resources tend to keep harmful bacteria in check, not least because they require other bacterial species to exist because biofilms are 'multi-species assemblages'. They can't do it on their own.

In a healthy mouth potentially harmful bacteria are present, but not in numbers that cause us any problems. It is when the ecological balance is disrupted that the problems start; by understanding what characterises a healthy ecosystem we can look for medical and lifestyle interventions that promote health.[6] Currently, most attention is focused on the link between bacteria and our back plumbing, which returns us to sitting on the toilet considering our poo . . .

Bad guts?

Of course, when things go wrong with your back plumbing it's rarely a laughing matter. I say rarely, but erratic, explosive and extravagant bowel movements have probably always been amusing to those not suffering from them. Perhaps one day in a cave somewhere we'll find a stone-age cartoon daubed on the wall, hopefully in a colour other than brown, depicting some unfortunate early man not quite making it to the bushes in time. However, despite the potential for comedy, many modern humans are ravaged by a range of bowel conditions that make the simple act of eating and going to the toilet a constant, painful and sometimes humiliating torment. The big three are Crohn's disease and ulcerative colitis (UC) – together known as the inflammatory bowel diseases or IBD – and irritable bowel syndrome (IBS).

IBS causes a range of unpleasant symptoms including abdominal pain, diarrhoea, constipation, bloating and tenesmus, which is the rather pleasing word for the very displeasing feeling of incomplete evacuation. Crohn's and UC are similar in some respects and both can cause abdominal pain, bloody diarrhoea (as in diarrhoea with blood in) and weight loss. The main difference is that UC affects the colon, the large and final part of the intestine, causing ulcers to develop, while Crohn's can affect the entire gastrointestinal tract, striking anywhere from mouth to anus.[7]

What is interesting is that all three conditions are far from resolved medically, but in all three, and Crohn's and UC especially, the problem might not be with us at all. The problem seems to be linked with bacteria that live in (and on) us in such high numbers that their cells collectively outnumber our own by ten to one. We'll return to these hidden passengers, and our poo, in far more depth in later chapters, but first we need to consider the idea that gut diseases are on the rise.

Are gut diseases really becoming more common?

We need to put the statement 'seem to be getting more common' on a firm scientific footing before we start groping around for answers to the big question of *why* they should be getting more common. To do that requires that we take a short excursion into the science of epidemiology and the field of medical statistics. It will involve a little light number work, but nothing too strenuous, and armed with this knowledge you will be better equipped to deal with the baffling array of numbers that accompany medical stories in the media.

Prevalence

If we want to gauge the extent of a condition within a population, then we are generally interested in that condition's *prevalence*. This is a measure of what proportion of a population has the condition of interest at a given point in time. You'll note the careful use of the indefinite article for population: it's *a* population rather than *the* population, because the total human global population is in reality subdivided into many different subpopulations with fairly limited movement between them. This matters when it comes to calculating the prevalence of diseases. To take a reasonably extreme example, the prevalence of HIV in Botswana in adults aged 19–49 is estimated to be 23.4%, or nearly one in four. In the UK it is only 0.2–0.3% – that's one in 330 or more.[8] Many conditions are rather uncommon, so percentages (per 100 people) are not always that useful. Consequently, prevalence is often stated as the number per 10,000 or 100,000. If we average disease prevalence around the world (*the* population), then the number we come up with probably masks interesting and medically relevant local variation. This variation is not just geographical but might include differences between males and females, between ethnic groups or between different age groups. So, if someone reports the prevalence of a condition without further qualification, you should exercise some sensible caution in interpreting that figure.

Also note that the prevalence is by definition the proportion of people affected at a *given time*. That means the prevalence today may not be the same as the prevalence tomorrow or yesterday if affected people die or more people get the disease. Prevalence is, or rather should be, a snapshot proportion of those affected within a specified population and used correctly it is a very useful measure of how widespread a condition is within that population.

Incidence

The other number used to quantify diseases or conditions is *incidence*. Often used interchangeably with prevalence, incidence is a more complex idea. Essentially, it is a measure of the risk of developing some condition within a given time period, but there are different ways to express this risk and this is where confusion can arise. Strictly, the incidence of a condition is the number of people developing it during a given time period within a specified population. This is usually expressed as an incidence proportion, and it all get a little complicated. It's easier to understand with a hypothetical example (see box).

Incidence is sometimes expressed as a rate: in other words,

Prevalence vs incidence

Let's say our population of interest is 10,000 people. Over a three-year period there are 100 *new* cases of the condition.

- The *incidence proportion* is 100 cases per 10,000 people over that period.
- If we divide everything by 100, we get one case per 100 people (or 1%).

This is obviously related in some way to the prevalence, but that relationship may not be clear cut.

Imagine a non-fatal and long-lasting disease (say it takes ten years to kill a person infected with it).

- Initially it spreads rapidly through a population.
- After five years, we work out how it spreads and advise people accordingly.

After seven years, that disease may have a *very high prevalence*, because those affected by it in the first five years are still alive but...

...in years six and seven (after medical advice on reducing the risk of contracting it has been issued) the incidence might be *very low*.

new cases over time. In the case of our imaginary non-fatal and long-lasting disease above, if the incidence proportion in the two years following medical advice to stop its spread was 104 new cases per 10,000 people, then the incidence rate is 52 cases per 10,000 person-years. Dividing by time is useful because it allows diseases and conditions to be compared, just as expressing proportions as percentages makes it easier to get a handle on what's going on.

Incidence rate is not without problems. For example, it assumes that the incidence rate is constant over the time in which it is calculated, which may not be the case. In our imaginary disease it may be that the medical advice issued at the end of year five took a while to get through to the population and that the biggest effect on incidence came in the following year. Just as prevalence can mask some important subtleties, so too can incidence and it is best to be cautious when considering either number. To be honest, when the media use numbers in medical stories, it is best just to be cautious.[9]

The problem of 'artefacts'

Another reason for caution, and not just with medical statistics, is the complication of *artefacts*. Artefacts are unintended "man-made" factors that affect an outcome and a common factor that can cause an increase in a given disease is simply increased diagnosis of that disease. Maybe if you had had symptoms of IBS or Crohn's disease

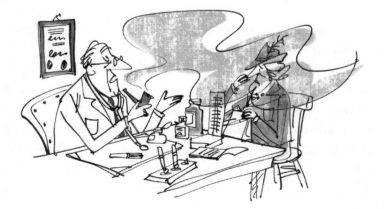

in the 1940s and you had gone to the doctor, he would have told you, through the haze of doctor-approved cigarette smoke, to get some fresh air and walk it off.

Attention deficit hyperactivity disorder (ADHD) was first described in 1902,[10] but when I was at primary school in the early 1980s not a single child had ADHD as diagnosed by a doctor. However, it is clear with hindsight that several 'naughty', inattentive children would be diagnosed with ADHD were they to present to a doctor today. ADHD shows an increase in prevalence over the last 40 years, but does this mean something important has changed with the mental health of our children, or that more parents are more likely to seek an ADHD diagnosis and doctors more likely to give one? Of course, a further complication here is that the answer might well include a bit of both.

The increased diagnosis artefact is always difficult to account for because there are so many factors that can have an influence on both sides of the doctor–patient relationship. Perhaps people are more likely to go to the doctor with potentially embarrassing bottom-related problems than they were? Maybe doctors are more likely to refer such patients to specialists who are more likely to diagnose? With the rise of the internet-informed self-physician, perhaps patients are more likely to self-diagnose and then push doctors towards that diagnosis?

What we really mean when we ask whether diseases like Crohn's are getting more common is: are they increasing in prevalence proportion and incidence rate and, if they are, is that increase because of some underlying change in our lifestyle or is it due to an artefact, most probably because such conditions are more readily recognised and diagnoses more likely to be made?

The rise of IBD is real

Factors like increased diagnosis have a role to play if we are comparing prevalence and incidence now with 50 years ago, or between the developed and developing world, but the more we compare like with like (small time scales, similar economic development and so on) the less important these factors become. However, even allowing for potential diagnostic artefacts, it is now widely accepted that inflammatory bowel diseases (like Crohn's disease and ulcerative colitis) have increased, and in many places are still increasing, in prevalence. Typically, in North America and Europe the number of new cases now is about double that of the 1950s and increasing trends have been seen virtually worldwide.[11]

Some countries are affected more than others. Scotland, New Zealand, Canada, France, the Netherlands and Scandinavia have the highest incidence and there is a link to industrialised status and affluence. So, does being rich cause Crohn's? Sadly it isn't as simple as that. Showing that one thing changes in relation to another is demonstrating what is called a *correlation*. Correlations are interesting and often very useful but they don't show that one thing *causes* the other.

Bacteria – the answer to everything? Maybe...

IBD is on the rise. As we'll see, other conditions and diseases are on the rise too, such as allergies, eczema, asthma, obesity and even depression. Science has started to reveal the key role that 'our' bacteria have to play in these conditions and how our lifestyles are damaging that relationship to our detriment.[12]

Throughout this book we'll explore how bacterial lives intersect with ours in fundamental ways that affect our health and well-being by means that we are only just beginning to fathom. It turns out that whether you are brushing your teeth, washing your hands, chopping chicken, suffering from an irritable bowel, battling with Crohn's disease, worrying about too little or too much hygiene, coping with asthma, breaking out in hives, stressing about your kids, cleaning your bathroom, flushing your toilet or guzzling probiotics, then bacteria are playing a central role in your life.

We will continue our journey through the human inner-ecosystem and discover the remarkable relationship between bacteria and our health in future chapters, but we have a complex relationship with bacteria in our homes too.

We were sitting on the toilet earlier and that's not a bad place to think about bacteria in a bit more depth . . .

CHAPTER TWO

'Kills 99% of Known Germs'

In which we consider everything you never wanted to know about the state of your toilet, via the cane toad, the power of bleach, the power of bacteria, how to protect yourself against faecal splashback – and whether any of it really matters.

Having spent some of the first chapter persuading you that bacteria 'aren't all bad', it's perhaps best to qualify that bacteria 'aren't all bad in the right place'. It's like oil. Wonderful stuff in a car engine but you wouldn't want to tread it across your carpet. Bacteria that might be useful in your gut, or the gut of some other animal, are far less welcome on the bathroom floor. Now, the whole concept of keeping a house 'too clean' and the notion of 'challenging your immune system' are topics for Chapter Nine, but let's be quite clear about one thing from the start. Widespread bacterial contamination of household surfaces is not a domestic arrangement that is sensitive to the development of little Johnny's immune system; it's a very real health hazard.

But if the bacteria in poo are 'ours', how can they hurt us? This is where thinking of our bodies as a complex ecosystem is especially helpful and a well-known case of organisms being in the wrong place is a helpful illustration of the point.

The cane toad
(just to be clear, not a bacterium . . .)

In the 1930s, Australian sugar-cane growers had a big problem with grey-backed cane beetles eating their crop. They are difficult to kill, but in Central and South America people had noticed that a big, no-nonsense amphibian, the cane toad, did a great job of eating similar beetles. As long ago as the early 1800s, cane toads had been introduced into the sugar-cane fields of Martinique and Barbados to control insect pests. By the early 1900s they were introduced to Puerto Rico and they were very successful in controlling cane beetles there. Spurred on by this success in the emerging area of biocontrol, thousands of young toads were released in Australia in the late 1930s.

Things did not run smoothly. Grey-backed beetles of Australia liked to hang out at the tops of the sugar cane, where big old cane toads couldn't climb up to reach them. Hungry cane toads, unable to pick off the plentiful beetles, started feeding on pretty much everything else instead, including some useful species that farmers wanted on their land. Toads also started poisoning the animals that tried to eat them, their warty skin glands being loaded with toxins. By voraciously eating the native fauna they also greatly reduced the food available for whatever species were left. Now there are 200 million of them, causing big problems by being in the wrong place.[1]

Bacteria that are present in our poo come from the lower end of our gastrointestinal tract. There, they are like cane toads in Panama or Venezuela: an established part of a stable ecosystem. The upper part of our gut, though, is a very different ecosystem, just as Australia is very different from Panama. There are different organisms living there, different bacterial communities and different environmental conditions. The cells that line that part of the gut are also different, with different genes being expressed and different products (like enzymes that aid in the digestion of food) being made. When we view our gut ecologically and from a bacterial point of view, it is not a uniform tube but a complex three-dimensional series of linked habitats. If bacteria from the lower gut end up somewhere else, then they are like cane toads in Australia, only instead of causing problems for the local wildlife, they can make us ill.

What can also make us ill, sometimes very ill indeed, are bacteria from the guts of other animals.

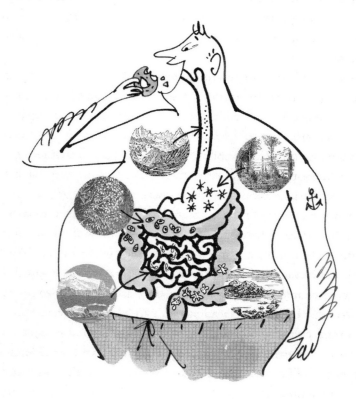

Burglary 101: seek out orifices

For bacteria to become a problem they have to enter our body and an obvious and very common route is through the mouth. In other words, we eat them, and that includes bacteria commonly found in poo as well as all the others you might find pretty much anywhere you touch.

You might not think of yourself as a *coprophage*, but you are. We all eat traces of poo if we touch surfaces that traces of poo have touched and then touch our mouths, or if we eat meals with 'poo garnish', added courtesy of poor food hygiene. In forensic science there's something called Locard's principle: every contact leaves a trace. The same principle applies equally in domestic hygiene, and the *faecal–oral highway* is by far the most common route for problematic bacteria from poo to enter our bodies.

The second common route is through another opening, the urethra, which is the hole through which urine appears. Bacteria from poo entering the urethra are the major cause of urinary tract infections (UTI). In both men and women the sewerage system for urine passes directly through what is also a 'recreational area', hence the joke about God being a civil engineer. However, in women the opening is much closer to the body, which makes it easier for bacteria from poo to enter. It's a simple geometry problem, really, but it's enhanced by other factors, most notably having sex.[2] Overall, studies indicate that as many as half of women will experience at least one UTI in their lifetime and some women suffer frequent UTIs. Displaced bacteria are the main cause, and an important culprit is *Escherichia coli*, or *E. coli*, a bacterial species found in the intestines of warm-blooded animals, including us. About 90% of UTIs and a significant proportion of gastroenteritis and food poisoning are caused by it.[3]

Faecal splatter

Once a poo is in the toilet neatly flushed away surely any contamination problem is dealt with? Well, not quite. For starters, that flushing action will have created thousands of tiny water droplets that become airborne, forming what physicists call an aerosol. Aerosolised water droplets contain bacteria from poo so, the next time you flush, close your mouth, keep your distance and shut the lid.[4]

It's obvious that poo-aerosols could land on surfaces close to the toilet and that touching those surfaces could result in poo-mouth transfer. It's also obvious that leaning open-mouthed over the bowl as you flush is a poor idea. It's less obvious that items left

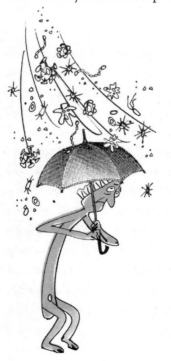

near a toilet can be contaminated, but official advice from organisations like the UK's National Health Service suggests we close toilet lids before flushing, and store toothbrushes upright, more than 2m from the bowl.[5] Studies also suggest that contact lenses could become contaminated if stored near a toilet.[6] It all starts to sound like the nanny state gone mad: even Mary Poppins never had a song about avoiding a pooey toothbrush. So, are we right to be paranoid about faecal aerosols?

The short answer is 'yes', with a longer answer being 'yes, a little bit, but don't be silly about it'. It is perfectly possible, and indeed simple, to test whether toothbrushes can and do become contaminated with bacteria from our guts when we flush. Various tests have set up artificial bathrooms, tested real bathrooms, tested brushes in all manner of different orientations and used simple agar plate culturing to find out what bacterial species occur, and they all come to the same conclusions. Objects in bathrooms get contaminated by bacteria that we can find in poo when we flush, but there's a big difference between poo on the bristles and a bout of gastroenteritis.

Just because we can culture *E. coli* from a toothbrush does not necessarily mean that we are going to fall ill after brushing our teeth. The presence of *E. coli* on surfaces and objects and in water (for example around beaches) is certainly an indication that those objects and places might have been contaminated with poo. However, most *E. coli* are harmless…

The reason that some *E. coli* are 'bad' and others are 'OK' is that bacteria are more than a little problematic when it comes to thinking about what we mean by a 'species'.

The problem of 'species'

We accept that all human beings on Earth are a single species and it is common knowledge that our species is called *Homo sapiens*, which means, however inappropriately, 'wise man'. However, some scientists studying our evolutionary origins argue that living human beings all belong to a subspecies called *Homo sapiens sapiens*: so good we named it twice. They would argue that Neanderthals are *Homo sapiens neanderthalensis*, in other words a subspecies of modern humans. Others say that they were an entirely separate species called *Homo neanderthalensis* and this argument seems to be winning at the moment. The point is this: the genus *Homo* is not diverse and, being our own, attracts considerable attention, yet there are still arguments raging over species and subspecies.

Many other organisms have subspecies identified within the 'main' species. For example, the cougars of the Americas (big cats, not sexually rapacious older women) have six subspecies living in different areas; the plains zebra of Africa has five. The minimum number of subspecies is, of course, two and we recognise a subspecies to be a group of organisms that could interbreed with other groups, the other subspecies, but that in nature don't, perhaps because of geographical isolation.

Subspecies cause all sorts of problems because it is actually very difficult to draw a line between them, even when the organisms are easy to study. Nonetheless, we recognise subspecies in a great many different organisms. In bacteria, we tend not to recognise subspecies but refer to strains instead. A strain is a genetic variant that has characteristics which distinguish it from other strains.

In the case of E. coli, a common bacterium associated with faecal contamination, there are a great many different strains. In fact, there more than a hundred recognised and that number is only likely to increase. What's more, bacterial species like Shigella (species of which cause dysentery) are now realised to be closely related to E. coli and would probably be better classified as part of the Escherichia group. Not only are there a great many different strains of E. coli, but many of those strains are not especially similar to each other. Only about a fifth of the genome is common to all strains, and some strains are so dissimilar that they should really be a different species.[7]

All in all, it's a bit of a mess. However, while its classification is far from straightforward, the fact that E. coli is the most studied bacterium means that we know a great deal about it, or, more accurately I guess, about them.

E. coli O157:H7:
definitely not 'friendly bacteria'

If you are keeping an eye out for bacteria-laden droplets escaping your toilet bowl, then I suggest you keep a particular look out for E. *coli* strain O157:H7. This is an especially unpleasant strain that causes haemorrhagic diarrhoea. Hard to spell, and harder to live with, haemorrhagic diarrhoea is both bloody and nasty, usually accompanied by severe abdominal cramps. Cows and sheep are the natural hosts for these gut-living bacteria, which most commonly get into us via infected beef.[8] Most people recover within a week or so, but around 5%, especially children under five and the elderly, develop haemolytic uraemic syndrome, in which red blood cells are destroyed and the kidneys fail. Without medical treatment, this is fatal and O157:H7 is the leading cause of renal failure in young children in the US.[9]

Why, then, are O157:H7 and other strains like O104:H4 (linked to a bacterial outbreak in Germany in 2011) so bad when strains like O150:H5 aren't? Why is it that some strains of E. *coli* cause no ill effects, some cause a 'bad tummy' and yet others can kill you?

Pathogenicity, the ability to cause disease, arises in O157:H5 because it produces a protein-based toxin called Shiga-like toxin, but before we find out how it managed to acquire such a toxin we need to consider some important biochemistry.

Make no mistake about it, proteins are very useful. Not only are they the structural components of tissues like muscle and skin, they are the molecules that form enzymes, the biological catalysts that control and orchestrate the multitude of chemical reactions that occur in our cells and help us to digest our food. Proteins form channels through the membranes that surround our cells and they can control the complex traffic flow of molecules in and out of those cells. They also make up the so-called cytoskeleton that gives our cells structure and provide internal 'tramways' for moving molecules around. So, proteins are very useful but they can also cause serious problems in the wrong place and in the wrong hands. For example, snakes and bees derive their venomous power from proteins.

What are proteins?

Proteins are long chains of smaller building blocks, called amino acids, which are joined together.

The order in which these amino acids are joined, and the overall length of the protein that they make, dictate the biological characteristics of that protein.

The 'letters' of the genetic code, the rungs in the twisted ladder of the DNA double helix, tell the machinery inside our cells the order in which to assemble amino acids in order to produce proteins.

Shiga toxins

Shiga-like toxins derive their name from shigellosis, a disease caused by infection with bacteria belonging to the genus *Shigella*. We met these bacteria earlier: they are the ones that cause dysentery and should probably be part of the *Escherichia* group. *Shigella* produces Shiga toxin, and O157:H7 produces a very similar toxin, which in *E. coli* is known, somewhat unimaginatively, as 'Shiga-like toxin'. Both Shiga and Shiga-like toxin act in a very similar way. Since we're talking about E. *coli*, it makes sense to focus on the Shiga-like toxin it produces, which, when we separate it from the bloody diarrhoea and suffering it causes, is a molecular wonder.

Shiga-like toxin is actually six subunits packaged up together. By weight, the subunit that causes the problems (the 'strike force') makes up just under half the toxin, and the remainder consists of five much smaller subunits that are the 'insertion team'. The toxin attacks tiny blood vessels in our gut. The smaller subunits attach to the outer parts of the membranes of cells that line these vessels and cause changes to the membrane that allow the toxin to be taken up. Once inside the cells, the larger subunit shuts down the cellular machinery for making proteins, killing those cells and preventing them from producing new ones. Since the tiny blood vessels are constantly renewing themselves, shutting down the cells' ability to make new cells causes the blood vessel to degenerate rapidly and to haemorrhage, hence the bloody diarrhoea.[10] So, how did some E. *coli* suddenly develop the molecular equivalent of an SAS unit?

The answer to that lies with viruses, specifically a group called *bacteriophages*. Viruses are little more than 'infective particles'. They have genetic material enclosed in a protective protein coat, but really nothing else. They are not cells and not normally considered to be living, although they do have some characteristics of living organisms, not least of which is the fact that they have genes and they reproduce. However, they lack any of the machinery required to read and make use of the genes encoded in their genomes. To do that, and to reproduce, viruses need to hijack the machinery of a cell. We are familiar with viruses that affect humans – HIV, Ebola and the common cold, for example – but bacteria can also become infected by viruses. Viruses that infect bacteria resemble a lunar

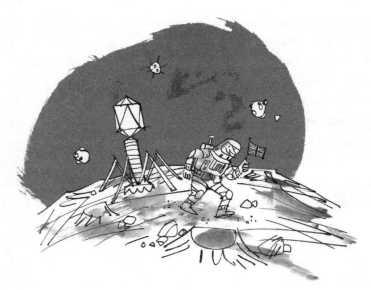

landing module and are called bacteriophages, or, if you want to be down with the lab kids, phages.

Phages are much smaller than bacterial cells and they inject their genetic material through the cell's outer membrane with a mechanism that is best described as a molecular hypodermic syringe. Once inside the cell, the bacterial machinery starts to translate the virus's genetic code and manufacture proteins, thereby making new phages. In hijacking the cell, the newly created phage can also acquire some components of that cell's DNA through a variety of different mechanisms. In a sense, the virus can become 'infected' with genes from its host and the nature of the bacterial genome makes this much more likely. If those genes prove to be useful for the phage, then phages carrying them will reproduce at a faster rate than those that don't.

Transfer of genes between phages and bacteria isn't a one-way street. Just as phages can acquire genes from bacteria, bacteria can also acquire genes from phages that have, in turn, acquired those genes from other bacteria. Those genes can become integrated into the bacterial genome. This process is called *transduction* and results in something of the 'keys in the fruit bowl' approach to exchanging genetic material among bacteria. It means that bacteria can acquire new genes from other bacteria and can sometimes be producing proteins that are the consequence of phage genes rather than their own.

Deadly bean sprouts

The outbreak of E. coli in Europe in 2011 affected nearly 4,000 people and killed 53, of whom 51 were in Germany.[11] It was caused by strain O104:H4 and in some cases was traced to what seems like an innocuous source: bean sprouts. Eaten raw, some bean sprouts were contaminated with E. coli that, within its genome, contained phage genes coding for a Shiga toxin. Strain O157:H7 also has genes coding for Shiga toxin that it has acquired from phage infection. *Shigella*, of course, has genes that produce Shiga toxin and it is thought that transduction via phages caused those virulent genes to spread to other bacteria, including many strains of E. coli.[12]

Flush, don't eat

I'm painting a pretty horrific picture of faecal contamination, but it's noteworthy that some people do consume their own poo. It's not common, for sure, but *coprophagy* has long been associated with brain tumours, dementia, obsessive compulsive disorder and sexual fetishes. In most cases this is a repeated behaviour, so clearly ingesting a little poo hasn't harmed the eaters in any lasting way. Young children pick stuff up and eat it all the time and this inevitably means that they consume poo, often their own. Bear in mind also that the next time you brush your teeth (and very probably every other time too) you are probably transferring faecal-borne bacteria to your mouth.[13]

The scary nature of *E. coli* and other bacterial, poo-borne infections tends to lead us to think that every poo lurks in the toilet bowl ready to pounce on us and infect us with life-threatening bacteria, or to separate itself into thousands of microscopic droplets that carry themselves onto our toothbrushes and contact lenses. But remember, even *E. coli* has a great many non-pathogenic strains and a healthy person is not likely to be shedding pathogenic bacteria. You've been brushing your teeth with *E. coli*-contaminated brushes for most of your life. The problem is that sometimes people can appear healthy but be infected, and infected people displaying symptoms like vomiting and diarrhoea have had

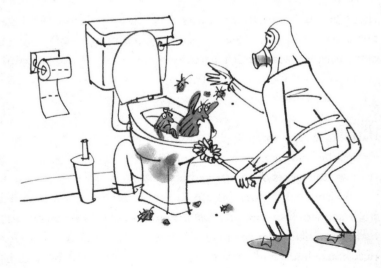

their bodily functions hijacked in a way that explodes bacteria all over their surroundings.

'Clean' isn't 'dead'

Diarrhoea, such as that caused by virulent *E. coli* infection, by *Shigella* or by *Salmonella*, can cause particular problems in the bathroom for three reasons. First, it is likely to be loaded with the bacteria that caused the problem in the first place. Second, genuinely 'explosive' diarrhoea leaves a toilet bowl and sometimes the area around it, looking like a poo-bomb has gone off. It gets everywhere and this makes it difficult to clean up and easy to come into contact with. The same rules apply to vomit, which is often projected with such force that splatter is unavoidable.

The third reason is that sometimes infective bacteria in faeces can persist for a remarkably long time in the environment. *Salmonella* is a gut-living bacterium, found in a number of animals, that can cause serious health problems in humans. Salmonellosis is characterised by diarrhoea, fever, vomiting and abdominal cramps and is very unpleasant. If a particular strain spreads to the lymph system, then things can turn truly nasty and cause typhoid fever and death if not treated. Incorrectly prepared pork, poultry and fish, where preparation has allowed gut contents to contaminate the meat, is commonly to blame for outbreaks, but the most severe strain, the one that leads to typhoid fever, is usually contracted through the faeces of an infected person.

A study of households in which a member had suffered from salmonellosis found that four out of six households still had *Salmonella* under the toilet bowl rim even after cleaning, that two households had a persistent biofilm containing *Salmonella* under the water line and one had it present even four weeks after contamination.[14] The bacteria were only found in wet areas, so the top of the seat and the flush handle were clear, but in and around the toilet bowl were far from clear, even though cleaning products had been used. So, if you are gung-ho about toilet hygiene most of the time, maybe be a little more careful if someone in your house is actually ill or if they are infected but not showing symptoms. Of course, that might make them rather hard to spot.

How can toilet cleaners not kill the one thing you really want them to kill?!

Perhaps the most disturbing feature of the study of *Salmonella* persistence is that pathogenic bacteria can live in toilet bowls for a long time, despite those toilets being cleaned. Is *Salmonella* not included in the 99% or 99.9% of germs that disinfectants are supposed to kill? Or is it that disinfectants don't really work outside of the laboratory?

The issue here is not that disinfectants don't 'work'. They do. In fact, many are very effective indeed at killing bacteria. There's a whole range of different disinfectants that we can use to tackle bacteria in our toilet bowls, but among the most commonly used are those based on bleaches. Many commonly available household bleaches are based on compounds containing chlorine, generally as sodium hypochlorite. Another familiar bleach is hydrogen peroxide, used extensively in hospitals and for turning your hair a lighter colour. They both work by attacking molecules on the outside of the bacterial cell membranes and causing the bacterial cells to die. Specifically, they attack proteins and, rather as boiling an egg turns liquid proteins into solid proteins, bleach causes proteins to lose their structure and function as they aggregate into insoluble clumps, killing the cells. They have the same effect on our proteins, which is why gloves aren't such a bad idea when you are handling bleach.[15]

It's not quite as simple as 'bleach kills bacteria', actually. In high concentrations that is certainly the case, but at low levels some bacteria have a way of resisting the seemingly irresistible chemical onslaught. Proteins are very big molecules and to work properly they have to fold up correctly to make a molecule that has the right shape. Some proteins form subunits that aggregate together to form what are termed oligomeric structures (we met one of these earlier – Shiga toxin): they need to be prevented from forming incorrect structures and encouraged into forming useful ones. Guiding proteins to ensure that they fold and group correctly is the role of molecular chaperones, which are, you've guessed it, proteins that assist in all this protein choreography.

Most of the early chaperones studied were involved with preserving protein structure when cells were exposed to elevated temperatures and they were termed heat-shock proteins or HSPs. But there are HSPs that respond to other stressors. HSP33 is one such chaperone. Found in bacterial cells, HSP33 activity responds to changes in how oxidising or reducing the environment is. Oxidation and reduction in chemistry are to do with losing or gaining electrons and it is oxidation that is at the heart of what bleaches do to proteins on and in bacteria. In oxidising conditions (like when bleach is added to the toilet bowl), some new chemical bonds form in HSP33 and it changes its shape, and its function. Suddenly (and these things happen quickly) HSP33 chaperone function is 'turned on' and it protects other proteins from the harmful oxidative environment. Of course, this only helps up to a point. HSP33 has evolved in the natural environment and we are capable of producing an oxidative environment far more brutal than most bacteria will ever have been exposed to.[16] What HSP33 teaches us is that if you are going to bleach a toilet, don't dilute it. Go in strong.

Other oxidising agents are used in disinfectants. Iodine is used in the poultry industry, ozone is used to disinfect water (along with chloramine and chlorine dioxide, giving swimming pools their distinctive smell) and potassium permanganate is sometimes used to disinfect feet before entering swimming pools.

Not all disinfectants work by oxidation. Para-chloro-meta-xylenol, PCMX, better known as the main ingredient in liquid Dettol, messes with proteins on bacterial cell membranes, causing cells to leak and let PCMX in to wreak more havoc inside the cell. Alcohol, mostly ethanol, is also sometimes used to disinfect surfaces, although it is more commonly used to disinfect hands – or to intoxicate. Like PCMX, it attacks cell membranes, this time dissolving the fatty component and messing around with protein structure, which is worth thinking about when you next drink the stuff.

Disinfectants like bleach, PCMX and ethanol have a very broad killing spectrum. They operate on aspects of fundamental chemistry that are vital for cell function. In a sense, there's nothing 'clever' about them and this sledgehammer effect has meant that these disinfectants are used the world over.

Why don't disinfectants always work?

Cleaning complex objects like toilets, and the sort of complicated three-dimensional surfaces we tend to have in our bathrooms, is actually really difficult. It's remarkably easy to miss parts of the toilet, to get bored and generally to do a bad job. Studies of home cleaning are not especially high on the research agenda but, not surprisingly, hospital cleaning practices have been subject to some rigorous examination. In one such study, researchers assessed surfaces in a patient's room for bacteria and for the presence of ATP, a compound found in all living material and one that is often used as a measure of 'biological contamination'. ATP readings showed that surfaces were cleaner after being cleaned (although not entirely clear of ATP), but that nearly a quarter of surfaces had bacteria present and that two especially notorious antibiotic-resistant strains were still holding on. Bear in mind this was a study in a private hospital and the surfaces being examined were pretty easy to clean. They were grab rails, bedside rails, remote controls and half the toilet seat. They weren't getting in around the bowl, or rooting out poo-ey residue from under the seat hinges following an attack of splatter-guts.[17]

Secondly, I suspect that we aren't always applying sufficient disinfectant for long enough. A quick squirt around the bowl and a quick flush, or a cursory wipe with a cloth containing already diluted disinfectant isn't likely to result in the bacteria-apocalypse you had planned. There's a relationship between the concentration and the contact time required for disinfectants: reducing the concentration increases the time you need to be disinfecting. Sometimes that relationship isn't straightforward. Phenol solution, or carbolic acid, was widely used in the 20th century as an antiseptic and is the active ingredient in many oral sprays used to numb sore throats. Halving its concentration increases the time required by a factor of 64. This is why following instructions is such a good idea. Trying to eke out disinfectant by diluting it or simply not mixing it up in the right concentration very likely means that it is not working as well as it should.

Have bacteria got the upper hand?

It is tempting to say that a third reason that disinfectants don't always work is that bacteria have got the upper hand. We have already seen that HSP33 might afford some bacteria protection against weak bleach and it is common to find articles and claims online that bacteria have developed resistance against disinfectants. Let's stamp on that claim right now. Bacteria have evolved resistance in some cases to certain antibiotics, but antibiotics are drugs that we take (or give to animals) and they are very different from disinfectants like bleach. If we think of a bacterial cell as being like a house, then antibiotics are like gentlemen cat-burglars, using skill and sophistication to gain entry by picking a lock or climbing through a tiny fanlight window. Bacteria can develop better locks or ways to keep their windows shut and we'll find out more about how they evolve resistance to antibiotics in Chapter Five.

Disinfectants are less like a cat burglar and more like a full-on meteorite strike. It doesn't matter how well the house is put together, what fancy locks are installed or how proficient your bricklayer was, the whole thing will be reduced to rubble in the base of a massive crater if the meteorite is big enough, or the disinfectant concentrated enough and applied for long enough. As we'll see, the evolution of resistance requires that some bacteria (maybe only one) can survive the initial strike and produce offspring bacteria that inherit the genes that allowed their parents to survive. There is no way for some bacteria to resist such a full-on strike, because it attacks the fundamental chemistry on which life is based. A truly bleach-resistant bacterium would be a very different bacterium indeed from anything we have seen anywhere in the living world.

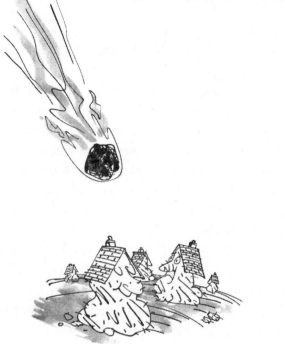

That said, some bacteria can produce bacterial spores and these are very tricky to kill. *Clostridium* species like *C. botulinum* and *C. difficile*, as well as *Bacillus anthrax* (the clue to its notoriety is in its name), are such bacteria. These species can form what are called *endospores*. Essentially smaller, simplified, toughened-up versions of the bacterial cell, endospores can survive in a dormant state and are able to withstand the onslaught of detergents and even alcohol. What they can't survive is bleach, but they need long contact times with strong solutions to ensure they are destroyed.

Bacteria biofilms, introduced in Chapter One, can also help bacteria to withstand disinfectants. They can be physically and chemically protected by the substances they produce that keep the cells together in a biofilm. But guess what? Bleach can get through if it's given enough time and it's sufficiently concentrated.

Other bacteria, the *mycobacteria*, have a waxy cell wall that means they can withstand the action of many disinfectants. These are the closest we have to 'disinfectant-resistant' bacteria and, given that both leprosy and tuberculosis (TB) are caused by mycobacteria, they are more than just a laboratory curiosity. Even though such bacteria can withstand prolonged exposure to all manner of chemical onslaughts, and are naturally resistant to some antibiotics, including penicillin, good old bleach will still do the trick, although concentration and exposure time are as important as ever. Recent work has shown that acetic acid, which is basically vinegar, is also effective, and far more user-friendly than bleach.[18] So, even problematic bacteria can be killed with the right disinfectant applied in the correct way.

The problem is that the real world isn't a lab experiment and factors like difficult-to-clean surfaces, the availability of disinfectant, the knowledge and ability to mix at the right concentrations, the time to apply disinfectant for long enough and the fact that cleaning is really boring all play a part in making disinfection practice less effective. The thing is, most of the research out there is, for obvious reasons, dealing with hospitals and really nasty bacteria. In reality, are you that worried about leprosy or TB in your bathroom? Even bacteria like *Salmonella* and Shiga toxin-producing *E. coli* strains aren't really a problem for the vast majority of us virtually all of the time. In fact, most of the time, most of the bacteria in and around our toilet are probably not going to do us too much harm because they are non-pathogenic. What's more, the chance of us ingesting sufficient numbers to cause any problems is extremely low – as long we aren't doing something stupid, like eating diarrhoea or making a habit of licking our toilet bowls.

Sitting back down

Let's go back to thinking about sitting on the toilet. Poo is released and it falls into the water. Some splashback might occur and this is a feasible way for bacteria to enter the urinary tract or to end up on the buttocks and later be ingested. However, the first depth charge is falling into clean water, which would tend to reduce the problem of bacterially contaminated splashback considerably.

US Patent US6170092 B1

Fear of faecal splashback was a revelation to me, but it seems that at least one person has already patented an idea to reduce it, albeit against a background of desperately ill-informed AIDS paranoia.

US patent US6170092 B1 is for a splashback toilet guard to 'protect a person from AIDS-contaminated toilet water that can splash back when Bowel Movements are made'.

The applicant confuses HIV (the virus) with AIDS (the disease) but ignoring that, and the fact that toilet splashback is not a causal factor in becoming infected by HIV, the device in question is simply a toilet-paper pad with polystyrene chips inside it that floats on the surface. You can examine the patent here: http://www.google.co.uk/patents/US6170092

I would suggest it's unlikely that you will be issued with a cease and desist notice if you use a wadded-up pad of toilet paper to achieve the same effect. That is, if splashback is something you fear. Personally, I think of it as a cheap bidet . . .

Once the offending item is dispatched into the bowl, there then follows some wiping; contaminating your hand with faeces is certainly feasible, and even quite likely with low-quality toilet paper. However, careful washing of your hands afterwards, using good old hot water and soap as we shall see in Chapter Four, is going to take care of any bacteria there.

Then you lower the lid (gentlemen, this means that you avoid all those tiresome toilet-seat conversations) and flush it away. In other words, the poo *was in the toilet* and now *it's not in the toilet*. Not only has it disappeared, but the toilet is now more or less sealed. Bacteria are far less likely to have aerosolised onto anything, and any that are left can't escape. Bacteria in the water can't fly out of the water unless the water is disturbed. So, as long as you don't lick the toilet bowl or drink the water, *they can't get you*! Chuck some bleach down there or use a toilet cleaner that releases all the time and you are doubly protected.

But, I hear you say, what about public toilets and door handles? Or public toilet taps? Or, for that matter, the taps and door handles in my own house? What if someone with *Salmonella* or some other diarrhoea-inducing bacterial infection has a faecal Niagara in the toilet, doesn't wash their hands and then touches the door handles? This seems like a reasonable concern, but let's break it down.

Don't panic

Firstly, most of the time most people don't have diarrhoea or some other transmissible infection. Secondly, when they do, they are most often at home, locked in a toilet. Very few people venture out. Thirdly, not all diarrhoea is caused by transmissible bacteria.

In a study of people with diarrhoea in Indonesia (where the consequences can be a little more serious than just a torrid time on the toilet), it was found that only 9% of 6,760 patients had diarrhoea caused by bacteria. Many (48.6%) of these cases were caused by *Shigella* (in other words bacterial dysentery), and *Salmonella* accounted for 29%. Both these bacteria cause diarrhoea in the UK; however, the fact we have access to good sanitation means that what we might consider 'common' is in reality rather rare. In 2013 there were 1,822 cases of bacterial dysentery reported in England and Wales, although the actual number is likely to be higher because many cases go unreported.[19] Just to put that in perspective, against a population of about 64 million people in 2013, that's really not that many cases. It's one in 35,126 people. This is about the same odds as tossing a coin and getting 15 consecutive heads (or tails, which seems more appropriate for some reason). The odds may not be as favourable for some sectors of the population. Extensive travel to developing world countries, or being a sexually active gay man, increases the chances of contracting *Shigella*, but even then bacterial dysentery is not exactly an everyday event. *Salmonella* is a lot more common but there were only 7,585 confirmed cases in England and Wales in 2013.[20] That's one in 8,437 people, or about the same odds as tossing a coin and getting 13 consecutive tails.

Overall, the chances of there being pathogenic bacteria on your door handles are really very small. Even in a public toilet the chances are low, but clearly increased by the volume of traffic. On top of the overall low risk, an infectious person has to not wash their hands correctly (although admittedly that applies to more than 70% of us, as we'll see in Chapter Four), the bacteria have to live long enough on the dry, hard metal surface to infect you (in practice many species don't thrive on such surfaces) and then you have to touch the right part of the handle, ideally with wet hands (to aid transfer), pick up the bacteria and transfer them to your mouth in sufficient numbers to become infected. I'm not saying it can't happen. Unlikely events happen all the time because of the sheer number of people, but it starts to look like something that shouldn't keep you up at night. That's really my point. We don't need to be paranoid about bacteria; just careful. If you are concerned, use your elbow to open the door. Just don't lick it afterwards.

So, remember, in theory, poo is harmful but it seems the greatest risk is of contracting a UTI, which is not what most people fear when they worry about toilet hygiene. Of course, poo *might* contain bacteria that *could* be very harmful indeed and *even* cause death. However, in all likelihood it almost certainly doesn't.

As if to prove the point, people eat the stuff all the time. Some children practically live on it if the alarmed questions on parent internet forums are to be believed. If you're worrying about eating poo accidentally, then it pays to remember the excellent advice given by the Illinois Poison Center of the USA on the subject of 'my child has eaten poop': 'Ingestion of a mouthful amount … is not considered toxic.'[21]

Sensible (one might even say obvious) safeguards mean you're probably not going to come into contact with bacteria from poo and, even if you do, you can wash your hands. Assuming you are reading this in the developed world you are extremely fortunate. You have a 'smallest room' with a toilet and a good sewerage system. So stop worrying and enjoy the peace and quiet that this set-up affords. That said, if the toilet does looks like a poo-bomb has gone off in it, then it might be wise to find somewhere else for a period of quiet contemplation.

CHAPTER THREE

If You Can't Stand the Heat ...

In which we consider the multitude of bacteria in our kitchen and their cunning tricks, why we shouldn't panic about most of them, why we should be very careful about others, and why we should always cook chicken. We also meet the world's luckiest melon farmers.

After the bathroom, the room of the house with the most obvious connection to bacteria is the kitchen. If our main concern is ingesting them, then the room where we prepare food is an obvious port of call. Back in Chapter One I urged you to think ecologically about the bacteria in your gut, to think of that great fleshy sewerage pipe as a complex, connected ecosystem. Such an approach is also useful when thinking about your kitchen.

First, think about the complexity of the physical environment in there. There is a wonderful array of tiling, grout lines, crevices, worktops, shelves and flooring in which bacteria can live. All these different habitats offer a full menu of choices. Don't like it too wet – no problem, move into this worktop crevice here. Like it moist and warm – hey, that dishwasher seal looks perfect. The bathroom is all hard, smooth porcelain: a desert in comparison to the warm, moist woodland of the kitchen. Not only is the physical environment welcomingly diverse, there is a wealth of material to consume. Bacteria in the toilet have a relatively limited diet; those in the kitchen have a choice of pretty much everything we eat, as well as all the bits and pieces we don't.

On top of all this habitat and nutritional diversity, we also have a regular re-introduction programme. Through this well-established and well-funded route we add population to the bacteria species already there and we introduce some new species to set up outposts in our kitchen. We call it shopping, and every time we bring back fresh fruit, vegetables and raw meat we add to the ecosystem already established.

567,845 bacteria per square inch!

It's really no surprise that bacteria should be present in colossal numbers in our kitchens. It is very easy to find alarmist media stories taking the 'latest research' and spewing out numbers that make your eyes bleed thinking about them. For example, there are, apparently, '567,845 bacteria per square inch' in your kitchen drain[1] (that's 88,016 per square centimetre if you prefer to work in metric), although what a square inch of drain actually means is hard to say and, let's be quite clear, that number is wonderfully but pointlessly precise. Also, I don't eat from my kitchen drain, nor do I use it in the preparation of food. If a recipe tells me to marinate something, my first instinct is not to stuff it down the drain and pour on the sauce. I'd be as bold as to assert that I couldn't care less about what lives in my drain.

It gets worse – 10 million per square inch!

567,845 is a big number for sure, but how about ten million bacteria per square inch on a kitchen sponge, which apparently is 200,000 times dirtier than your toilet?[2] Ten million is a lot, right? I mean that's a sixth of the human population of the UK and more than the population of 42 of the 50 states of the US. And that's just in a square inch (about 6.5 square centimetres) of kitchen sponge. If we scaled that up then we could be talking billions of bacteria in our kitchen. Well, yes; trillions.

But what does any of this mean? Without knowing what species are present, and how abundant the harmful ones are, these abstract 'large numbers' are just plain spurious. They seem terrifying, but bacteria are very tiny and large numbers are something they do rather well. There could be 40 million bacteria in a gram of soil, yet we don't see horror headlines telling us to stay out of the garden. In fact, as we'll see in Chapter Nine, we might actually be healthier if we had spent more time in our gardens. We need to dissect these shock headlines and find out what species and strains are present, assess whether they are potentially harmful, determine whether they are simply present or if they are abundant, work out if we are actually likely to ingest any of them and then decide if there might be something obvious and simple we can do to mitigate that risk. In short, we need to be a bit more rational about the whole thing.

Let's start with the source of all kitchen scare stories, the dirty germ-bomb, the apocalyptic source of certain death that is the kitchen sponge. The kitchen sponge regularly tops the bacteria charts, at least in the tabloid press, and if you prefer a more retro approach to your dishwashing then be assured that the dishcloth doesn't fare any better. These things are covered in bacteria. But think about it – of course they are. With their tremendous surface area, near-constant humid environment and regular replenishment with food fragments, it's hardly surprising that bacteria thrive there. That doesn't mean they are a health hazard.

There have been a number of studies of cloths and sponges used in dishwashing and the findings aren't as clear-cut as you might think. Some studies fail to find anything of much concern, but one showed that 37% of dishcloths were infected with *Listeria*, including the species that causes us harm, *Listeria monocytogenes*.[3] This sounds truly dreadful. *Listeria* is nasty. It causes listeriosis and the elderly, the newborn and pregnant women are particularly at risk. *Listeria* infection can be fatal. Most people infected in the UK are hospitalised and approximately one-third die. Make no mistake about it, *Listeria* is a serious thing. So, given that one study showed that 37% of dishcloths had *Listeria*, then surely this must be a major public-health hazard? I don't understand how we are still here as a species. Is it only people who use dishwashers who survived the great sponge purge? WHY DOESN'T THE GOVERNMENT DO SOMETHING, FOR PITY'S SAKE!!! Also, why don't I know a single person who has ever had it?

Listeria hysteria

The reason we aren't all dropping like flies is that while *Listeria* is common, listeriosis is not. The number of cases in the UK every year is consistently in the low hundreds. The Centers for Disease Control and Prevention (CDC) in the US estimates the incidence of listeriosis to be just 0.26 cases per 100,000 people in 2013.[4] It's serious, yes, but it's not common.

Microbiologists describe *Listeria* (the bacterium, remember, not the disease it causes) as 'widely distributed', which in microbiological circles tends to mean 'where we look, we find'. In terms of the sort of thing we might find in our kitchen it is most commonly associated with soft cheeses like Brie and Camembert (which is why pregnant women are advised to give these a miss), but it has also been found in pâtés, butter, ice cream, sliced meats, poultry, smoked salmon, packaged sandwiches, unpasteurised milk, canned fish and unwashed fruit and vegetables. It also does pretty well at low temperatures, which is a bit of a problem given that the fridge and freezer are our stock responses to slowing down bacterial growth. It has been isolated in water, soil, vegetation, processed food, a variety of mammals, birds, fish, insects, the poo of domestic animals and us. In fact, according to one study it can be found in the poo of more than 60% of apparently healthy people, so there's not a bad chance that you have it dwelling within your gut right now (although reported percentages vary from less than 1% up to 70% in laboratory workers handling *Listeria monocytogenes*).[5]

The reason you probably don't have listeriosis right now is that either you don't have it in your system or that your immune system is mounting a robust response to it. *Listeria monocytogenes* produces a molecule (a protein yet again) called an invasin that allows it to get into cells, including the macrophage ('big eater') cells of our immune system and cells of the gut wall. Once inside these cells, the bacteria can multiply and move around the body, potentially causing 'problems' or, to put it more medically, listeriosis.

Part of a healthy immune system is called cell-mediated immunity or CMI and it is our CMI that kicks in when *Listeria* invades. Special cells, called T cells, can identify *Listeria* and destroy it before it can cause a problem. Most healthy people, with a healthy immune system, may experience some symptoms if the infection gets going a little, typically like mild influenza, but normally the CMI does its job and *Listeria* doesn't get too far past the front door.

The problem arises when it hits someone with a compromised immune system, when the CMI can't keep it at bay, although even apparently healthy people can sometimes be affected.[6]

The world's deadliest melons

Listeria outbreaks, when a large number of people are infected, are far from common but when they occur they are serious. A particularly nasty outbreak, highlighting that *Listeria* isn't just found in unpasteurised dairy or processed food, occurred in the US in 2011. The culprit or, more accurately, culprits were cantaloupe melons. Eventually traced to a specific supplier, Jensen Farms Colorado, the melons caused listeriosis in well over 100 people in multiple states and killed 33. It was the third-deadliest food outbreak in US history and it was caused by a combination of easily preventable failings at the melon-packing plant. The floor was poorly maintained, while dripping water from a condensation line was allowed to pool on the floor, leading to *Listeria* growth and contamination of equipment that wasn't cleaned properly. Inspectors also found a second-hand potato-cleaning machine being used to scrub the melons, which, unless they grow very small melons or very large potatoes in Colorado, doesn't seem like a good solution. The brothers who owned and ran the farm were prosecuted and found guilty of causing the outbreak, although they avoided any jail time because of a 'lack of intent'. Reading the facts of the case it is hard not to think that either they were very lucky or they had acquired the services of the sort of lawyer you definitely want on your side.[7]

So, should we be concerned about *Listeria*? Yes of course we should, but that concern should be rational, and directed towards the real hazard. What are you more likely to get *Listeria* from – a dishwashing sponge or infected food? Or, to put it another way, an object you don't eat that may (but also very well may not) have *Listeria* on it in relatively small numbers, or something that is the ideal breeding ground for *Listeria*, that carelessness in food preparation could infect and that is bought for the sole purpose of eating? *Listeria* outbreaks are rare and that's largely thanks to stringent food-preparation rules. But, as the Colorado melon outbreak teaches us, mistakes can happen and, when they do, the results can be fatal. Health and safety legislation is not just about some spoilsport stopping you from setting up that chainsaw-juggling children's entertainment business.

On the other hand, scare stories about terrifying bacteria lurking in seemingly innocuous places around our homes, workplaces, health clubs, pub toilets and virtually any other private and public space are mainly a result of us being able to investigate such places more easily and cheaply than we could before, and bothering to do so. The presence of bacterial species that can be pathogenic doesn't mean that we should cordon off the kitchen and starve or, sadly, stop going to work.

But back to the kitchen and to the other great source of media panic when it comes to 'harbouring killer germs': the chopping board. Like many of us, chopping boards start off life smooth and blemish-free but with use the surface becomes scarred and pitted. Couple all those lovely bacteria hidey-holes with the fact that many of us probably use the same chopping board to prepare pretty much all food (albeit with a quick wipe down between courses) and we clearly have an ideal contamination and infection station.

Next time you make dinner . . .

By now you will have seen the pattern emerging, so I'll cut straight to the chase. Studies of chopping boards have shown the presence of *Listeria*, *Salmonella*, *Campylobacter* and our old friend from the bathroom, *E. coli* (not necessarily from our poo, as we'll see). Now, while 'finding bacteria on things' doesn't equate to 'people dying in droves', even a back-of-the-envelope analysis and a bit of common sense tells us that chopping boards are something we should be a little bit careful with. I invite you to join me in preparing a meal. Nothing fancy, obviously: not on an academic's salary.

Let's make a nice chicken dish. Perhaps a bit of chicken breast (with a helping of *Campylobacter* and a splash of *Salmonella*) pan-fried in some cream (side order of *Listeria*) with some leeks (a bit of *E. coli* to garnish) and mashed potato on the side, a few herbs stirred in, maybe? Glass of wine in the sauce, the rest for me. Official story: 'Mosht of it went in the schhauce . . .'

Here we go. First I pour a glass of wine to get the creative juices flowing and then I take the chicken out of the fridge. I always mean to buy from a nice local butcher, but the fact is it's tricky to park so today's chicken is in a wrapped plastic tray with some kind of 'conscience-logo' suggesting that the former possessor of these fine breasts didn't live a completely awful life. I grab the first knife that comes to hand, the standard short kitchen knife (I'll need that later, too) and I run the blade around the thin film restraining my breasts. The glass of wine means my hand is not as steady as I'd like and I graze one of the breasts, but it doesn't look serious. They get tipped on the board and I cut out the weird little mini-breasts (cunningly marketed in the US as chicken tenders) with a sharper knife to save for my kids. Put both

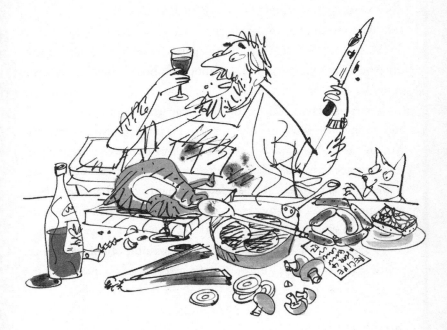

knives on the board and have another glass of Riesling. Breasts go in the pan with a bit of oil. OK, time for veg.

Potatoes are going to be peeled and boiled for mash, so I won't bother with any chopping-board-cleaning nonsense. Twenty minutes in boiling water will kill any bacteria, so a quick peel and chop and they're in the pan, with a sneaky top-up of my wine glass. Time to start on the other veg, so I'll turn the board over, thereby using the clean side. Clever!

Another top-up, then chop the leeks. This little knife is rubbish, so the sharp knife gets an outing. I'm partial to a bit of raw leek, so a cheeky chef's treat and then into the pan they go. Chopping board ends up on the floor as I transfer the ingredients, but I'm pretty sure it landed chicken side up, which saves me from floor-cleaning detail. Quick toilet break and I think my wife's saying has the chopping board had chicken on it? 'Not on that side, darling,' I shout, somewhat louder than the 'I think' that comes after.

Back down to the kitchen and it's time to get the breasts out of the pan. I'll plonk them on the chopping board for now. I assume my wife didn't flip it . . .

It's very easy, even with the best intentions, to end up contaminating surfaces like chopping boards and worktops. Knives touch raw chicken and get put down on chopping boards that people assume are clean but aren't, then you forget which side is which or which board was used for what. I love raw vegetables and my habit of taking 'chef's treats' doesn't help the contamination issue. Given all this activity, it's not at all surprising that bacteria are readily found on such surfaces. But, as always, we need to address the key question – is it actually a health hazard?

Salmonella

Let's focus on *Salmonella*, which is certainly a bacterium of concern when it comes to food preparation. Like *E. coli*, *Salmonella* is diverse, with a large number of different strains as well as some different species. Some cause typhoid fever that, like listeriosis, happens when the infecting bacteria travel away from the gut and start to infect the rest of the body. Typhoid fever occurs when you ingest food or water contaminated with the poo of someone with typhoid fever and is predominantly a disease of the developing world. It reflects inadequate sanitation and poor food and water hygiene. A far more likely scenario in the developed world is that a person becomes infected with a non-typhoidal strain of *Salmonella*, which can result in the aptly named salmonellosis.

So, how does *Salmonella* end up on our food? Well, like most of what we've met so far, *Salmonella* is a gut microbe and it's found in the guts of a large number of domestic, wild and farmed animals. When meat is prepared, great care is usually taken to ensure that gut contents don't come into contact with the meat. Sometimes not enough care is taken and the problem is that contaminated meat (which includes pork, beef, chicken and seafood) quite likely looks and smells fine. Animal poo can contaminate our food by another more direct route. It can end up tainting fruit and vegetables because irrigation water is contaminated or perhaps because animals poo directly on the crops, which then find their way into our fridges and mouths. Seafood can be contaminated if the water in which it lives is contaminated. *Escherichia coli* from mammals and birds, including dangerous strains, find their way into our gut via the same routes. It's because of this animal connection that salmonellosis is sometimes referred to as a *zoonosis*, that is, a disease transmitted to humans by animals.

Once in our gut, *Salmonella* gets to work. For anything between 12 hours and a few days it multiplies quietly in the intestine, then the trouble starts. *Salmonella* invades the cells of the gut wall in a similar way to other pathogenic bacteria, including some *E. coli*.

The inside of our gut is lined with epithelial cells and each of those cells (and indeed every cell) has a cell membrane. This fatty wonder of molecular architecture keeps a cell together and is the connection between the inside of the cell and the rest of the world. A *Salmonella* bacterium attaches to the cell membrane and on the bacterial cell membrane are special protein assemblies called Type III Secretion Systems or injectisomes. They work rather like a syringe, injecting so-called effector proteins into the cell that cause an effect (proteins are often aptly named) in the host cell. In the case of *Salmonella* that effect is quite dramatic. Affected epithelial cells are triggered to extend their membrane outwards, forming a kind of membranous pocket that engulfs the bacterium and brings it inside the cell in a neat little cell-membrane bag.[8]

Normally this process works out pretty poorly for anything potentially harmful that finds itself dragged into a cell. Special tiny 'bags' called lysosomes, full of enzymes, fuse with the bacterial bag (more properly called a vacuole) and fairly quickly digest whatever is inside. But, cunningly, *Salmonella* injects a second protein and this causes changes in the vacuole membrane that prevents the lysosomes from fusing. Once inside the cell the *Salmonella* bacteria wreaks havoc, resulting in abdominal cramps caused by inflammation, bloody and mucous diarrhoea, elevated temperature: in fact, all the symptoms that very soon confirm you have food poisoning.

Listeriosis is unusual but salmonellosis is more common and, like listeriosis, can be associated with outbreaks as well as isolated incidents. Eggs are one source of *Salmonella* since the shell exterior can become contaminated with chicken poo, and bacteria can then infect the interior. The US Food and Drug Administration (FDA) estimates that 142,000 people a year in the US are infected with *Salmonella* from eggs.[9] That's a lot of bloody diarrhoea, but it is possible to protect the public from at least one source of *Salmonella* (see box).

Despite the fall in overall cases of *Salmonella* in the UK, there are still outbreaks and often there's not a chicken in sight. In 2014, for example, there were a number of clustered outbreaks in the UK, with 32 cases associated with a Chinese restaurant in Hampshire, 31 linked to a Chinese takeaway in Merseyside, and, lest we think that by avoiding Chinese food we'll stay safe, 34 cases associated with the Birmingham Heartlands Hospital.[10]

Take egg-ceptional care ...

In the UK a famous political storm broke out in 1988 when government minister Edwina Currie announced that most of the UK's egg production was infected. This sparked a massive downturn in egg sales and a furore that rapidly led to her resignation, and a whole carton-full of egg-stremely dreadful puns in the nation's press.

In 2001, details emerged that there had been something of a cover-up and that while Currie's pronouncement that 'most' of the UK's eggs were affected had been a little enthusiastic, the general sentiment was spot on.[11]

Since 1998, UK eggs branded with the Red Lion mark have been produced by chickens that are vaccinated against *Salmonella* and the number of reported verified cases of salmonellosis in the UK has dropped and continues to fall. The total in 2013, according to UK government data, was 7,585 cases, compared to nearly double that in 2001. The vaccination of hens is probably the biggest factor in this decline.[12]

Sometimes rather a lot of people can succumb. The 2013 Street Spice festival in Newcastle led to 413 people feeling spicier than they might like after uncooked curry leaves left them suffering from diarrhoea and vomiting. *Salmonella*, *E. coli* and *Shigella* (yup – that's bacterial dysentery on the streets of the UK) were identified from several, but by no means all, of the sufferers.[13] Some people had more than one bacterial infection at once, which seems especially unlucky, although no one died as a consequence of the outbreak. Should this put you off street food?

Not necessarily, but it is clearly reassuring if you can buy food that you can actually see being taken out of scalding oil or from a bubbling pot.

The Night (on the toilet) of the Iguana

It's not just infected food that can lead to salmonellosis. If you are the sort of person who likes to keep reptiles or amphibians, then handle them with care. Not only can Iggy the iguana give you a pretty impressive nip but, like other lizards, snakes, frogs, toads, tortoises, turtles and terrapins, his excrement can carry a hefty dose of *Salmonella* transferred out from his natural gut microbiota. Handling these animals, or dealing with the water from their tanks, can lead to infection.

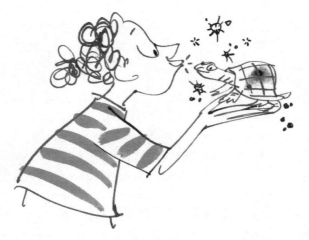

Small children are especially vulnerable. In the US between 2011 and 2013 there were eight *Salmonella* outbreaks affecting

473 people across 41 states, as well as Washington DC and Puerto Rico. Nobody died, but 29% of the sufferers were hospitalised and these cases were traced back to 'exposure to turtles and their environments'. Of those affected, the median age was four. The median is a type of average that works by lining up your data points (in this case the ages of each person affected) in rank order (lowest to highest) and working out the 'middle' value. In these outbreaks such a low median is a very strong indicator that young children are being unusually affected: a statistical inference supported by the fact that 31% of cases were in children below the age of one, and 70% in those under ten.

Why are children so vulnerable? It's largely because of a behavioural pattern we've already encountered: they put stuff in their mouths. This is a useful habit when it comes to feeding, but sadly the stuff they shove in there is not always beneficial. Sometimes it's a small toy, sometimes it's a lump of poo and sometimes it's Thomas the terrapin. The link between *Salmonella* and turtles small enough to fit into an inquisitive child's mouth is so well established that the FDA has a regulation that specifically bans the sale of live turtles, terrapins and tortoises less than 4in (10cm) long. Title 21, Chapter 1, Subchapter L, Part 1240, Subpart D, Section 1240.62 (I'm not making this up), or the '4-inch rule' (named for the size of chelonian it bans rather than its typed length), has been in place since 1975; breaking the rule carries a potential one-year jail term and a thousand-dollar fine.[14]

E. coli . . . again!

We've already met another potentially pathogenic bacterium, *E. coli*, when we were in the bathroom, which seemed like a good place to introduce this most studied of all bacteria and best known of all the gut microbiota. However, as we saw, it is only some strains that cause us any real problems and of those some are especially notable. The most common way for E. coli to enter our system is not by the direct human faecal-oral route that we all fear (although clearly this can happen), but by a more indirect animal poo-oral route. I took a look at the list provided by the Centers for Disease Control and Prevention (CDC) of outbreaks in the US and here are some of the sources: raw clover sprouts; ground beef; ready-to-eat salad; organic spinach; raw clover sprouts (again: note to self, avoid clover sprouts...); in-shell hazelnuts; romaine lettuce; cookie dough; pizza; fresh spinach; and a travelling petting zoo in Minnesota.[15]

I think when most people think 'food poisoning' they tend to think 'meat', especially perhaps chicken (and for good reason, as we'll see), but many E. coli outbreaks are associated with salad and vegetables. What is more, many of them involve O157:H7, the nasty strain that produces Shiga toxin. And be assured, in every case someone has ingested those E. coli, which means that they have eaten animal or possibly human poo. Of course, not all poo on our food is infected, so you could argue that at least those people who got ill knew they'd eaten it. Most of us, most of the time, just munch away on it without realising. Not much comfort, to be honest.

Chicken . . . bacterial roulette?

I'm going to be spending most of the remaining chapters of this book trying to convince you that bacteria are mostly either harmless or beneficial, but since we're trawling the high-profile glamorous end of the bacterial beauty show, the pathogens, and since the chicken dinner I started earlier is rapidly cooling down, it feels like the right time to introduce a real player in the world of food poisoning and one that doesn't always get the public recognition it deserves. *Listeria* rhymes with hysteria, so that's the press coverage sorted even for the laziest headline writer; *Salmonella* has real brand recognition; and *E. coli* has a suitably 'sciency' ring to it to appeal to editors. *Campylobacter*, on the other hand, is tricky to spell and sounds like an ill-conceived and effeminate cycling accessory.

Despite its relatively low level brand awareness, *Campylobacter* is the cause of a great deal of gastroenteritis, which is the medical term for all the abdominal pain, diarrhoea and vomiting we have been encountering so far. In fact, in the developed world, campylobacteriosis is the leading cause of bacterial gastroenteritis, causing an estimated 280,000 cases a year in the UK alone, with 65,032 cases positively identified in England and Wales by the Health Protection Agency in 2012.[16]

Campylobacter is notable for having an exceptionally rare but potentially very serious complication. Since the almost complete elimination of poliomyelitis, the most common cause of acute neuromuscular paralysis in the world is Guillain-Barré Syndrome (GBS). GBS occurs when the immune system gets a bit confused and starts to attack the wrong thing, in this case the nervous system. It is an autoimmune disease and we will encounter more of these in later chapters. It can be treated, and 80% of sufferers make a full recovery, but there can be long-term problems with mobility, sensation, balance and strength in those who don't.[17]

About 60% of GBS cases occur after viral or bacterial infection, which seems to trigger the immune system to attack nerves. Cases can develop as a consequence of gastrointestinal infections and one of the most commonly associated is *Campylobacter*.

A recent systematic review of the published literature from around the world concluded that 31% of GBS cases are attributable to *Campylobacter* infection,[18] but let's be honest: a much more pertinent statistic is what proportion of people with campylobacteriosis are likely to end up with GBS? The same systematic review estimates that between 30.4 and 117 cases of GBS develop per 100,000 cases of *Campylobacter* infection. In the UK it is estimated that there are 1,200 cases of GBS a year, which, again with some back-of-the-envelope calculations, means that 372 might be attributable to *Campylobacter*, working out at just under 133 cases of GBS per 100,000 infected. Even if we take the higher end of the estimates, GBS is still a rare complication.

The leading way for *Campylobacter* to get into our system is poultry. About 50% of cases arise from handling and eating poultry, although you can also become infected from eating pork or beef, drinking unpasteurised milk or contaminated water (meaning water with animal poo in it) or by having contact with pets and farm animals.[19]

Why it is advisable to keep your mouth shut if you're looking up

Campylobacter means 'curved bacteria' and there are a number of different species of this distinctive, corkscrew-shaped bacterium. The species that cause most of the infections in humans are *Campylobacter jejuni* and *C. coli*, not to be confused with *E. coli* (the jejunum is the name given to the middle section of the small intestine, whereas *coli* refers to the colon or the lower gut). *Campylobacter jejuni* is the star of the show, though, causing more than 85% of infections in humans, and is the species most commonly associated with GBS. Generally found in poultry, it also occurs quite naturally and generally quite harmlessly in the guts of other birds, including wild birds. One study showed that just under one-third of wild starlings in Europe shed C. *jejuni* in their poo, which is something to consider if you ever go to watch a murmuration.[20] These great assemblages of thousands of birds wheeling the autumn sky are amazing to watch but, on the ground, are characterised by two sensory experiences that the TV coverage doesn't really convey. First, they are incredibly noisy and second, you are subjected to a rain of poo if they happen to be 'murmurating' overhead. It makes me wonder how many chicken dinners are falsely blamed for a dose of the runs when the real reason might be more complex. I don't think that should put you off watching birds, but I do advise keeping your mouth shut if you're looking up.

Let's be sensible . . .

The problem with the modern world of instant media and constant news is that it provides the perfect nurturing environment for the sort of paranoia that is entirely natural but easily encouraged to grow beyond the point where it is helpful. A gung-ho approach to kitchen hygiene will end in tears. Actually, it will likely end in liquid flowing from another part of your anatomy that will need more than a tissue to clear up. The simple fact is that some of the food we eat is contaminated with bacteria. This isn't a 'fault' of the food industry per se, although clearly there are measures that can be, and in general are, taken to reduce this contamination. We are animals eating other animals and plants that have had contact with the environment and with animals and their products. Those animals have within them ecosystems with inhabitants that do not fit in our internal ecosystem. Whether those undesired passengers hitch a lift on meat and poultry or on fruit and vegetables, there are some simple (in fact, let's be honest, common sense) things we can do to reduce the risk.

The first, most obvious thing to do is to stop worrying too much about side issues. Bacterial gastroenteritis outbreaks do not occur because some journalist reports that your kitchen drain has *Salmonella* living it. Think through the risks sensibly and remember that bacteria are everywhere and if we look we often find. Very few species can harm us and just because these potential pathogens are present doesn't mean that we are going to come into contact with them, or that they are present in sufficient numbers to be a concern.

Kitchen sponges can be contaminated, at least according to some studies, and clearly using a sponge covered in potentially pathogenic bacteria and using it to wipe those bacteria over surfaces and dishes is a bad idea. But it doesn't need to be treated like some kind of spongy psychopath trying to wipe out your family. If you are worried, then dipping your sponge in a solution of bleach is a very cheap and easy way to disinfect it, and it's also a good idea to get rid of sponges before they get too scuzzy. Wringing it out thoroughly and letting it air-dry after use will help with hygiene. Bacteria grow best in moist environments and will struggle in drier sponges. Don't use it on food. Don't clean off your chicken with it, don't polish your pumpkin with it and don't use it to buff up your broccoli. Oh, and finally, don't eat it. It's not that kind of sponge.

Some bacterial species like *Salmonella*, *Listeria*, *E. coli* and *Campylobacter* can cause food poisoning, but the clue as to how you are overwhelmingly likely to get infected by them is really in their colloquial name – *food* poisoning. It is food, and food preparation, that we need to worry about most in our homes. Modern techniques in farming and food preparation lessen the risks we face and have undoubtedly played a substantial role in the large reduction we have seen in cases of some bacterial food poisoning over the last 20 years or so, but there is more that can be done. Mistakes still happen and while there's nothing we can really do before the food reaches us, once we have control we can take sensible precautions that don't mean we are being paranoid.

It seems sensible to consider chicken as being potentially contaminated because, at least in the UK at the moment, this is the simple fact. In a recent survey by the Food Standards Agency, 59% of shop-bought fresh chickens tested positive for *Campylobacter* and 16% of those tested at the highest level of contamination. *Campylobacter* is not just 'there': in many chickens it is present at a level that is not conducive to being away from the toilet for long. Although more stringent regulations in production will undoubtedly reduce this level over the coming years, it seems sensible to realise that about one in six chickens has really quite a lot of *Campylobacter* living within it.[21] Chicken eaters need not cast aside their Kievs in disgust, however. Here are the simple 'chicken rules' to avoid food poisoning.

1) *Absolutely do not wash raw chicken.* It splashes and aerosolises bacteria around your kitchen, it contaminates your sink and it achieves precisely nothing. Stop doing it.

2) Store raw chicken, covered, at the bottom of a cold fridge where it cannot drip on other food through some unseen hole in the packaging. This is obvious, really, but so easy to ignore in the heat of the battle that commences on the return from a big shop with an already full fridge.

3) If raw chicken touches other food that is not going to be thoroughly cooked straight away, then that food should be considered to be contaminated.

4) Utensils, surfaces and knives that touch raw chicken should be washed thoroughly. All that lovely steam in the dishwasher is perfect for utensils and a bit of bleach solution does wonders on your worktop.

5) Wash your hands properly with soap and warm water after handling raw chicken and dry them afterwards.

6) Cook it thoroughly – chicken is not a meat to be had rare on the basis of taste alone, never mind the bacterial aspect, so make sure it is steaming hot throughout, with no pink uncooked meat, and that the juices run clear. You could get a meat thermometer, but good luck with finding any consistent answer as to what temperature it should read. I can tell you that the highest internal temperature I've found suggested for whole chicken is 85°C throughout, and that will certainly do the trick. Others (the US CDC, for example) suggest 74°C, whereas the UK's Food Standards Agency goes for 'steaming hot throughout', which makes up in utility what it loses in precision.

Some more hygiene rules

Being careful around chicken is a pretty easy thing to do, but what about E. coli and its ability seemingly to infect everything from a salad sandwich to cookie dough? For advice there I turn to the CDC, because I reason that populations with a highly litigious reputation are likely to have official advice that is, at the very least, defensible in court. The CDC's advice is reassuringly sensible and easy to follow. In fact, it's pretty similar to the advice above. Wash your hands thoroughly after handling poo of any kind (going to the loo, changing nappies), after handling animals and before preparing food. Cook meat thoroughly and avoid cross-contamination by cleaning utensils and chopping boards. They also suggest avoiding unpasteurised milk, dairy products and fruit juices. Pasteurised are all fine – the process involves heat and that kills bacteria. Finally, don't swallow the water you swim in.[22]

The CDC also recommend washing fruit and vegetables, which, remember, are often implicated in E. coli outbreaks. The UK's NHS is just as forthright, and reminds readers that the 2011 outbreak in the UK, which affected 250 people, was probably caused by E. coli in soil stuck on the outside of leeks and potatoes.[23] The key thing here is to wash off the soil, which is where most bacteria are going to be. You aren't ever going to be able to wash off all the bacteria from the surface of an apple or a lettuce, but with a running tap and a good rub you can get rid of the soil sticking to your veg, and should get rid of most of the problem. A bit of dirt has limited nutritional value and likely comes from a farm environment with plenty of animal poo around. If you want to eat soil, then I'd suggest picking a source less likely to have animal gut microbiota as an added extra. Just a thought...

If you gather together all this advice you end up with some fairly simple rules that cover you for most bacterial eventualities. Avoid unpasteurised food, be careful of cross-contamination, wash your hands after handling potentially infected things and before preparing food, and keep your mouth shut when you don't need it to be open, which is actually pretty decent advice for many situations. Wash fruit and vegetables under a running tap and don't ever wash chicken.

The risk from bacteria in our food is real but, with care, that risk can be made really very small indeed. The problem is that even with simple things, like washing our own hands, it turns out we aren't very careful . . .

CHAPTER FOUR:

Why You Should Think Twice about Shaking Hands (Especially with Men)

In which we consider just how bad we are at washing our hands, how better hand-washing could save a million lives a year and how best to wash our hands, as well as whether we can get drunk on 'swine flu gel', while remembering that 'can' does not mean 'should'.

A common theme in the bathroom and the kitchen is the importance of something that has rather pompously become known as 'hand hygiene' but that most of us would regard as 'washing our hands'. If you look at a neural homunculus of a human being – those horrible disproportionate images of humans that represent body parts in terms of the proportion of the brain given over to them – then apart from enormous genitals the main things that stand out are massive hands and big lips. We are very manual–oral creatures and given that we touch our lips and shove stuff into our mouths frequently it is little surprise that bacteria on our hands can end up in our gut. It also therefore follows that washing bacteria off our hands is likely to reduce the chances of potentially harmful bacteria entering our system.

This isn't some ivory-towered conjecture. It has been estimated by the CDC, among other organisations, that poor hand hygiene contributes to 50% of all food-borne illness outbreaks and that hand-washing with soap could reduce diarrhoeal disease by more than 40%. Crunching the numbers leads to the somewhat shocking figure that better hand-washing could save one million lives a year.[1] Washing hands saves lives and it isn't brain surgery.

If it were brain surgery, though, we'd find hand hygiene to be considerably more detailed than most of us manage after a quick pit stop or a chicken-preparation session. If you watch a surgeon scrubbing up, you get a good idea of what hand hygiene is really all about. Careful washing of all hand surfaces, each individual finger, the wrist area, paying close attention to the palms and the backs of the hand as well as to the finger webs. This is a serious water-soap-hand ballet and my guess is that very few of us have ever washed our hands 'properly' and almost none of us wash them properly on a regular basis. Actually, it's not just a guess.

There's a little demonstration that I've often done at science festivals on hand hygiene, or the lack of it. I get people to apply a gel to their hands that is colourless but that glows eerily under UV light.[2] After the gel is applied I ask the people to wash it off. Washed hands then go into a light box and, sure enough, they have glowing patches in all sorts of places where the gel has remained. It's a nice party trick and a good demonstration of how ineffective hand-washing tends to be, but it isn't scientific and it doesn't measure bacterial contamination. To do that requires a larger scale approach, some old-fashioned observation (which can become legally problematic in public conveniences) and some bacterial culturing of unwashed and washed hands.

Washing your hands

Before tearing apart our collective hand hygiene it is worth
considering the proper technique, as provided by 'Wash your
Hands', a hand-hygiene campaign in partnership with the UK's
National Health Service[3]. As well as being genuinely useful
information, it also introduces the key components to a proper
hand-wash – water, soap, rubbing, rinsing, drying and time . . .

- Wet hands with water
- Apply enough soap or handwash to cover all hand
  surfaces, then rub as follows:
  o Hands palm to palm
  o Right palm over other hand with interlaced fingers and
    vice versa
  o Palm to palm with fingers interlaced
  o Backs of fingers to opposing palms with fingers
    interlocked
  o Rotational rubbing of left thumb clasped in right palm
    and vice versa
  o Rotational rubbing, backwards and forwards, with clasped
    fingers of right hand in left palm and vice versa
- Rinse hands with water
- Dry thoroughly with towel

Duration of procedure: at least 15 seconds.

Why it's better to shake hands with a lady

Fortunately, there are plenty of scientific studies dedicated to
hand-washing. Many of them, for obvious reasons and as we saw
with studies of cleaning in Chapter Two, tackle hand hygiene

in hospitals and others are concerned with the effectiveness of different hand-washing products. The remainder tend to examine hand-washing practice in the general public and the facts and figures both support my general observations and make me think twice about shaking hands.

The overall finding of these studies is that we are very poor indeed at washing our hands but exceptionally good at lying about it. In recent surveys in the US, for example, 94–96% of those asked said that they consistently washed their hands after going to the toilet, but these were self-reported values. In studies where people are directly observed the level of hand-washing tends to be much lower. One study in 2003 found that only 61% of women and 37% of men actually washed their hands after using the toilet in a public convenience.[4] Let's just ponder those numbers for a while. Fewer than four in ten men washed their hands after going to the toilet. Sure, women are a little better, but they aren't exactly bathed in glory either.

Another study was somewhat more encouraging, finding that 90% washed their hands, but only 67% used soap, the rest going for the old 'rinse and shake' routine. The length of time spent hand-washing is also far from encouraging, with the same study showing that only 30% of people washed for longer than nine seconds, and 70% washed for less than eight seconds (which includes the 10% that didn't bother wasting time on hand-washing at all).[5] What's especially discouraging about these results is that, if we are being honest, they are exactly what we'd expect. If you think about washing your own hands, or watching someone else wash theirs, then four to five seconds feels about right.

Men washed for a little less time than women (though only 0.8 seconds less) but were over-represented in the 'didn't bother' group, with 15% of men not washing at all and 35% doing the rinse and shake. Just over half (and only just – 50.3%) washed with soap and water. Women fared far better, with only 7% not washing and 78% using soap and water.[6]

However, only 5% of people washed their hands for longer than 15 seconds, which is still five seconds shorter than the 20 seconds recommended by the US CDC, by health advisers in Canada and New Zealand, WHO and others. Nailing down the science behind this recommended duration is difficult. There are few studies examining the health impact of different durations and those that have looked at hand-washing duration have focused on total microbial load rather than on those bacteria likely to cause harm. There are also a great many potential confounding factors, such as size of hands, amount of soiling and the recent history of those hands (whether that be food preparation, bottom-wiping or nappy-changing, for example). The balance of the evidence suggests that longer is better, though, and that 15–30 seconds is a sensible time.[7] Overall it's fair to say that, at best, only one in 20 people you meet have washed their hands in anything like an effective manner. A more pessimistic, but arguably more realistic, interpretation would be that, in terms of effective bacterial removal, no one has washed their hands.

Interestingly, the likelihood of hand-washing can be influenced by the presence of signs telling us to do so, but not necessarily in the way we might want. Women are far more likely to be manipulated by such means than men, at least according to one study. Women leapt from 61% to 97% hand-washing when a sign was put up telling them to do so, but men actually declined from 37% to 35%.[8] Other studies end up with different numbers but the same pattern emerges: we don't wash our hands as much or for as long as we should if we are left to our own devices; and men are a lost cause.

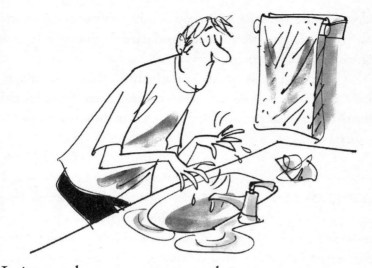

Is it ever better not to wash?

Not all hand-washing is equally effective. Just going through the motions after having a motion, with a quick rinse under a running tap and a shake-off, is no substitute for a proper wet, lather, scrub and rinse. Also, drying is very important because bacteria like moist surfaces and are more easily transferred from and to wet hands. This all seems quite straightforward and the advice is easy, at least in principle, to follow. The problems occur when the diversity of cleaning products, tap types and drying methods are thrown into the mix. Suddenly, washing your hands seems like a serious business and in some cases it can even seem as if you are better off not washing them at all.

The notion that you might be better off in some places not washing at all, perhaps because you suspect the water is unclean or the taps are filthy, is compounded by the fact that the 'punishment' for not washing your hands occurs a long time after the 'crime'. Bacterial gastroenteritis often takes a day or more to manifest itself following infection (and sometimes much longer), during which time plenty of food will have been consumed. Contaminated food has a much stronger and obvious link to a dodgy tummy, but the faecal–hand–oral route in the bathroom or the contaminated food–hand–oral route in the kitchen could play their part. So far, I haven't found a single study that suggests *not* washing your hands is a good thing.

Water, soap, rub, rinse . . .

Let's start our hand-hygiene analysis with the first thing you think of when washing virtually anything: water. It might seem that effective washing requires clean running water and certainly that would be a great start, but research has consistently shown that it is not essential. A study in an urban squatter settlement in Pakistan, for example (where water was faecally contaminated), provided one group of women with soap, a safe water vessel and the ability to sterilise water within it, and another group of women with soap alone. The 'soap only' group had to use untreated water to wash their hands. The research team made unannounced visits and tested the women's hands for faecally derived bacteria. They found that the two groups did not differ significantly and both had greatly reduced bacterial counts compared those who had not received soap. So, even dirty water can be effective in hand hygiene as long as soap is used.[9]

Another issue is whether the water should be cold, warm or as hot as you can stand. There's something very reassuring about the feel of hot water and soap on dirty hands, but it seems this is a purely psychological phenomenon. To kill bacteria through heat alone, the water would have to be far too hot for you to wash your hands comfortably, and although warm soapy water is considered to be more effective at removing oils that could hold bacteria from your skin, a number of studies have consistently shown that warm or hot water gives no improvement over cold.[10] What is more, heating up water to wash our hands simply wastes energy, produces more CO_2 and may even lead to increased skin irritation through the removal of natural oils. It is using soap and a thorough and vigorous scrubbing action that does the trick, rather than the temperature of the water.

Turning on taps is one part of the process that tends to make me think twice about washing my hands in what seems like a 'dirty' facility. You have to touch the taps with dry 'dirty' hands, and then again with wet 'clean' hands, just as everyone before you has done. At first sight it seems like the perfect bacterial transferral station and indeed WHO and others make recommendations to healthcare professionals to use a towel when operating taps (I presume a clean towel). Interestingly, though, I failed to find any data on whether taps are a source of re-contamination, which makes it hard to make an informed judgement. The generally cautious CDC agrees, and almost goes as far as to waggle a finger at those wasting paper towels to operate taps.[11] Using a paper towel to shield your hands from the taps will reduce bacterial transfer, but it is far from clear whether such bacterial transfer is a real hazard. The choice comes down to whether you think the cost to the environment of a paper towel outweighs the unproved benefit of using it. Personally, I don't use a paper towel to turn on taps, but to be honest that's because I don't wash my hands in the first place...

Let's assume we have clean running water pouring over our hands. The next step is the lather stage. Lathering assumes soap, but there are other cleaning products we'll examine in a moment.

Washing your hands with water alone and a good scrubbing action is actually better than nothing. In one study volunteers were required to touch door handles and railings in public spaces and were then allocated to one of three groups: no washing; washing with water only; and washing with conventional soap. Of the great unwashed 44% had faecally derived bacteria on their hands but only 23% of the water-only group were similarly contaminated, dropping to 8% in the soap and water group.[12] The reason why soap is so effective involves some basic chemistry.

Soap molecules are what physical chemists called 'polar'. This doesn't mean that they are cold. It means that they carry a tiny electric charge and in the case of soap also have two distinct 'ends', which are often known as the head and the tail. Think of it as looking a little like a molecular tadpole. The head end is a group of carbon, hydrogen and oxygen atoms arranged in a specific way that chemists call a carboxylate group. This head end carries a negative charge.

The head is negative because, like the stuff we put on chips (sodium chloride), soap is actually a salt. Chemically, this means that it is a combination of a metal atom (usually potassium or sodium) and a fatty acid. Because the potassium or sodium floats free of the head end when you add water, and because potassium and sodium carries a positive charge, it leaves a negatively charged head. The tail of the soapy tadpole is a long chain of carbon atoms linked together, with hydrogen atoms poking out down the sides. The crucial thing about the soap molecule – and indeed the molecules forming cell membranes, which are not dissimilar – is that the head end loves water (it is hydrophilic) and the tail end hates water (hydrophobic).

When soap molecules are put in water, the hydrophilic head ends interact with the water while the hydrophobic tails avoid it. This results in the spontaneous formation of minute soapy spheres called micelles, with the water-hating tails in the middle like the

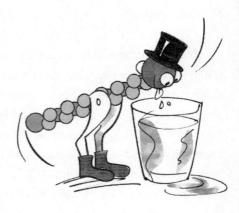

spokes in a three-dimensional wheel. Molecules that form grease and oil are hydrophobic like the spokes in the micelles, which is why water alone cannot disperse them. However, with soap added, the micelles trap the grease and oil (and anything else trapped in the grease and oil) and allow it to mix with the water, which then gets flushed down the sink. Conventional soap, then, doesn't kill bacteria, but it assists in dislodging bacterial biofilms and bacterial cells sticking to oils and grease on our skin.

The molecular action of soap is greatly enhanced by the physical action of scrubbing. Not only does this help to dislodge material clinging to our skin, it also helps to disperse the soap all over our hands and into the nooks and crannies where bacteria could thrive. After scrubbing, the hands should be rinsed to remove the dirt, grease and oil from them, as well as the bacteria that the physical scrubbing action and the chemical action of the soap have helped to lift from our skin. Running water is best for this and there's no reason for it to be anything other than cold water, thereby also saving energy. Everyone's a winner.

... and dry

Finally, the hands must be dried because bacteria can be transferred much more easily from and to wet hands. Now, you might think that drying your hands was a pretty uncontroversial side of the whole hand-hygiene topic, but you'd be wrong. Hand-drying is a multi-million-pound industry with a baffling range of products to choose from and ethical decisions to be made. Disposable paper towels or re-useable fabric towels? Or do you go down the electric air-dryer route and save hand towels? And, if you go electric, do you opt for hot air or a jet-like blast of cold air?

The evidence for the effectiveness of different hand-drying methods is horribly contradictory, with a multitude of biological, environmental and economic factors determining whether one particular method is better or worse than another. A clear and undisputed conclusion is that hand-drying is a 'good thing', but its role in hand hygiene has not received the same level of attention as other aspects, like the use of soap. However, a systematic review of what literature there is, published in 2012, examined a number of factors that contribute to the effectiveness of a hand-drying method. The review considered hand-drying in terms of drying efficiency, removal of bacteria and the potential for cross-infection.

Drying efficiency was measured in terms of the time taken to achieve a certain level of dryness, since all methods will ultimately dry your hands completely, given enough time. Indeed, provided you aren't in a 100% humidity environment, your hands will eventually dry themselves by evaporation, but in general we seek a rather quicker solution than that provided by ambient physics. Our usual methods either absorb water (cloth and paper towels) or act to speed up evaporation. This is achieved either by providing additional heat and removing water vapour via a fan or, in the case of many so-called jet-air dryers, simply by removing water vapour along with most of the higher frequencies of our hearing range.

The evidence for which method is the most efficient is reasonably clear. Cloth towels can reduce residual dryness to 4% in ten seconds and 1% in 15 seconds. A hot-air dryer takes about 45 seconds to get down to 3%, or 97% dryness if you prefer. However, a jet-air dryer in a different study achieved 90% dryness in ten seconds, which was an identical performance to a paper towel in the same study. So, if you want fast and efficient drying, then cloth and paper towels are excellent, jet-air dryers seem to be not too far behind and the old-fashioned hot-air dryer drags over the finishing line huffing and puffing long after everyone else has gone home. Even more supportive of the towel method is the fact that people are not especially inclined to spend long periods of time drying their hands in a public toilet. In one study, a hot-air dryer in a natural setting typically only achieved 55% dryness for men and 68% for women, the fairer sex displaying more patience yet again when it came to hand hygiene. Cloth and paper towels in the same setting achieved 90% or more in both sexes, showing the superiority of the towel method and that men are not incapable of hand-drying but, just as in other aspects of life, like to get the job done quickly.[13]

Bacterial removal is an interesting aspect of hand-drying because it may be that the action of drying your hands could add bacteria. Bacterial addition might occur from the material used to dry your hands or potentially from the electrical dryer unit itself. The weight of evidence here again leans towards the paper towel, with friction from rubbing against the skin helping to remove bacteria. Some studies have shown that hot-air dryers can add bacteria to the skin, although exactly how this happens is disputed. It may be contamination from the machines themselves or from some circulation of bacteria caused by the draught, as we'll see in a moment. In fact, the role of friction in removing bacteria from the skin is also poorly studied, but the overall conclusion, at least according to the most up-to-date review, is that drying hands with paper towels was the best means of removing bacteria from the hands.[14]

Finally, as we have already seen, bacterial aerosols from the toilet can spread bacteria around a bathroom, and so too can the air circulation caused by air dryers. As might be expected, some studies have indeed found that air dryers can disburse bacteria, from between 1m (hot air) and 'at least 2m' (jet air), and that paper towels produce negligible contamination. However, as you might now have come to expect, life is rarely that simple and sure enough other studies have found that air dryers cause no appreciable increase in contamination.

The overall conclusion is that paper towels are the best from a hygiene perspective and are recommended in hygiene-sensitive places like hospitals. However, air dryers do not come out of the study too badly and it's important to note that, as with a great many other hygiene studies, none of the studies of hand hygiene showed (or could show, given their methods) any actual link to diminished or increased human health. In other words, we don't know for sure whether much of this actually matters! We do know that infectious bacteria can be on our hands and that we can become infected, but whether using paper towels or a hot-air dryer and drying for 20 seconds rather than 15 seconds makes any real difference to health is not a question we can answer satisfactorily: we simply don't have a robust evidence base. I wouldn't let that put you off washing your hands, though, and maybe spend just a little more time doing it.

The rise of 'antibacs'

Before we leave hand hygiene, there is one more major issue that needs to be considered. So far, the assumption has been that if we are washing our hands at all then it involves conventional soap and water. This is not always the case and recently there has been a rise in two other hand-hygiene products that further muddy the waters of an already evidentially confusing topic: alcohol-based hand-sanitisers, and soap developed and marketed as 'antimicrobial', 'antibacterial' or, if you feel that 'terial' is just too time-consuming to say in the hectic modern world, 'antibac'.

There has been a similar glut of antibacterial products marketed for the kitchen, too, with antibacterial chopping boards being a prime example. In fact, even a casual perusal of the internet shows that just about anything that can be treated in order to make it antibacterial has been and is now available to anyone with a mouse button. There is a glut of different technologies out there, the details of many of which are difficult to come by, although some make use of silver (especially in textiles) and others use specific chemicals that discourage growth. Regardless of how they work, it seems likely that they do achieve at least some reduction in some bacteria. There is, of course, no evidence whatsoever that using such products has any effect on human health, though it seems likely that it could. Bear in mind, though, that just because you have bought a shiny new 'antibac' chopping board, you still shouldn't chop up raw chicken and then prepare a quick crudité on the same board. It is tempting to say that such products must have a beneficial effect on health even if it is small, but it is entirely possible that they could lead to complacency about basic hygiene and subsequent detrimental effects.

Up until a few years ago the only alcohol we got on our hands was from spilt drinks, but alcohol gels and other products for 'sanitising' hands are now so everyday that they regularly appear by the checkouts next to the chocolates and chewing gum. Alcohol has become synonymous with ethanol, which unless we are regular meths drinkers (meths being short for another alcohol called methanol) is the stuff that gets us drunk. Chemically, though, an alcohol is a molecule that contains carbon, hydrogen and oxygen, with one each of those oxygen and hydrogen atoms paired together in a way that gives the alcohols many of their chemical properties.

Many alcohols are very effective at killing some bacteria, with the alcohol dissolving the bacterial cell membranes and disrupting the proteins that cells rely on to function correctly. Incorporating the bactericidal capability of alcohols like ethanol or isopropanol within a gel that can be easily and conveniently applied to hands without the need for drying afterwards seems like the perfect solution to hand hygiene.

There is no doubt that sanitisers with an alcohol content of 60% or more (most are sold at around 62% or higher) are effective at killing bacteria on our hands. At around five times more alcohol content than wine, the ethanol-based products would also be very effective at getting us drunk, but the presence of a number of other substances reduces the appeal for most of us. Nonetheless, they are sometimes consumed and can lead to intoxication. One such case produced one of my all-time favourite headlines: 'Prisoner "drunk on swine flu gel"'.[15]

A wealth of studies, many based in healthcare settings, show that not only do alcohol sanitisers reduce bacterial load on hands, but they also do so, in many cases, with reduced levels of the skin dryness and irritation that can be associated with excessive use of soap and water.[16] Of course, in the ever-contradictory world of hand-hygiene research, there is also evidence that alcohol hand-sanitisers can cause skin irritation, but this can be reduced with various additives and, given the importance of hand hygiene in healthcare, further improvements will doubtless be made.

Alcohol is effective and that is why hospitals have hand-gel sanitising stations all over the place and signs requesting (and in some cases pretty much ordering) everyone to use them. They work, although so does soap and water and, against some bacteria, soap and water works better. Like soap and water, alcohol gels only work properly if they are applied properly, in the right quantity and for long enough. What's more, if your hands are heavily soiled, hand-sanitisers may not work as well as they should because they do not perform as well as soap in removing dirt, grime and grease. Yet again, the unavoidable conclusion is that unless you need to wash your hands all the time, and few of us do, soap and water still seem like the winning combination.[17]

There are also studies of non-alcohol-based sanitising gels, some carried out in schools where the presence of large quantities of alcohol in the form of not-quite-set jelly has an understandable lack of appeal. These products can contain a variety of antibacterial substances such as benzalkonium chloride (widely used as antimicrobial agent in the food industry). Interestingly, in a research sphere dogged by a lack of link between observed bacterial loads and measurable health benefits, at least one study has shown that using these hand-sanitisers might lead to reduced absences from school. However, such studies are always hampered by the ethical difficulty of having control groups and being able to take account of the many factors of complex everyday life that interfere with neat experimental designs; care therefore needs to be taken in interpreting such results.[18] Again, though, I haven't come across any studies suggesting hand hygiene is a bad thing.

Triclosan

There is one aspect of hand hygiene that might just be a 'bad thing' and explaining why requires us to consider a substance commonly used in non-alcohol antibacterial hand-sanitisers and in antibacterial soaps and handwashes: triclosan. Visually a rather pleasing molecule, triclosan is formed by a pair of hexagonal rings of six carbon atoms linked by a bridging oxygen atom, with two chlorine and some hydrogen atoms attached to one ring, and a chlorine atom and an alcohol group attached to the other. As a molecule it has a lot going on and some maintain that atomic symmetry and complexity lead to it having antibacterial properties.

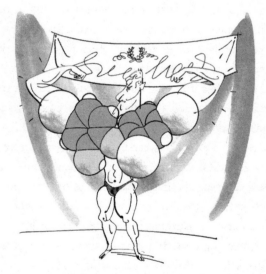

At low concentrations triclosan is bacteriostatic, which is to say that it doesn't do enough to kill but it prevents what is there from multiplying. At higher concentrations it can and does kill many but not all bacteria. It does its antibacterial work by binding with an enzyme that is essential in maintaining and building cell membranes. With triclosan bound to it, the enzyme no longer works, leading to cell membranes becoming destabilised and new ones unable to be formed.

Triclosan was used throughout the 1970s in hospitals, but since then it has been widely added to antibacterial soaps, handwashes, hand-sanitising gels, toothpastes, shampoos, shower gels, kitchen utensils, bedding, rubbish bags: basically pretty much everything that can be sold to people concerned about bacteria. In hospital environments throughout the world it is used in medical devices and as a body wash to eliminate troublesome bacteria like MRSA. In the home, as we've seen, good old soap and water, maybe a bit of bleach, and some sensible home husbandry is more than sufficient in most cases and extensive use of triclosan feels like overkill. In fact, it may even be overkill in hospitals as well: research to show whether triclosan handwashes or soaps are any more effective than soap and water is, you've guessed it, far from clear. In fact, the US FDA is involved in an ongoing regulatory review of triclosan, stating that 'the agency does not have evidence that triclosan in antibacterial soaps and body washes provides any benefit over washing with regular soap and water'.[19] The state of Minnesota has gone one step further, banning the use of triclosan in most retail consumer hygiene products from 2017. The EU has forbidden its use in food-contacting items since 2010 and in 2014 voted to ban it from disinfectants and a number of textile-based products.[20] Other authorities and countries (for example, Canada) look likely to follow suit.

Why are people so down on this attractive and effective molecule? The first problem, as the FDA has pointed out, is that there is no convincing evidence that it is of any use. This is not the same as saying it doesn't work. Triclosan most certainly does kill bacteria, but coating every surface and textile with it, sticking it in toothpaste, shower gel and countless other products doesn't necessarily result in better public health and in this case the evidence is lacking. Another problem is that all this triclosan ends up in the environment, messing with the literally countless bacteria out there in the world either doing us no harm or, in some cases, being positively beneficial. Water pollution isn't just about killing fish. Bacteria are absolutely crucial in the wider ecosystem and pushing out tonnes of harmful chemicals with little or no proven benefit to us is very last century. Finally, triclosan has been implicated in a biological phenomenon that is, for very good reason, rarely out of the news: bacterial resistance.[21]

CHAPTER FIVE

Resistance Is not Useless

In which we consider the beautiful inevitability of evolution, the rise and rise of antibiotic resistance, bacterial 'special cuddles' and nanoexplosive buckybombs.

If we want to stop ourselves getting bacterial gastroenteritis then, sure, we can follow some very basic food and general hygiene rules, but what about tackling the problem at source? Why don't we simply kill off the pathogenic bacteria inside the animals we eat? If they aren't in the animals' guts, then they can't be in their poo and we can't ingest them. For that matter, why don't we eradicate all bacteria from our homes by using substances like triclosan combined with constant hand-washing and cleaning?

Such a wholesale approach to the domestic environment is not that far from what we have, at least collectively, attempted to do. Bleach, an extremely effective product against bacteria, is still there, but it's been joined by a dazzling and frankly confusing assortment of pimped-up cleaning products promising bacterial apocalypse, but with the gentle scent of delicate floral blossoms to accompany our microbial massacre. Moving away from the cupboard under the sink we have silver in our socks, triclosan in our rubbish bags and Microban on our chopping boards. It's fair to say that domestically we have done our absolute level best to eradicate bacteria. Interestingly, much of this effort seems to be focused on the 'consumer approach', where we venture out to the shops ever hopeful that some new product will save us from the bacterial horde while paying such little regard to washing our hands properly that we may as well not bother. Ever vigilant for labour- and time-saving opportunities, we scoff at those still stupid enough to bother washing their chopping board when some miracle molecule will sort out those loathsome little *Listeria*. Yet still we find bacteria everywhere.

Outside of our homes the 'root cause' approach has actually been very successful in some cases. As we saw in Chapter Three, in 1998 supermarkets in the UK started to buy eggs solely from hens that had been vaccinated against *Salmonella* and that intervention has seen a massive drop in the prevalence of salmonellosis in the UK both from eggs and from chicken meat itself.[1] Vaccination, in this case, works and both chicken- and egg-consumers should be thankful for it.

So why no vaccination programme against *Campylobacter*? It is, after all, the biggest cause of bacterial gastroenteritis in the developed world and chickens are the biggest source. Nail *Campylobacter* in chickens and the benefits would be immense. Research is certainly underway, but it's a difficult job to get a vaccine that works every time. Also, once such a vaccine is developed, it will need extensive testing and then, since it is entering the food chain, there are further complications. At the moment, the research literature is full of 'excellent candidates' and 'promising developments', but we aren't there yet.[2]

Out of the cruel world come . . . antibiotics!

Vaccinations are one way to reduce the bacterial load in animals, but another is to give them *antibiotics*. An antibiotic is basically any substance that is produced by a microorganism (bacterium or fungus) that inhibits the growth of, or kills, other microorganisms. The microbial world is full of such substances because at the micro-scale it is a cruel bacterium-eat-bacterium world.

Given a new ecological opportunity, a bacterium's best evolutionary bet is to divide rapidly and colonise as much space as possible. Make hay while the sun shines, except here the hay is more bacterial cells and the sun is the continuing existence of whatever potential food it has colonised.

A bacterium that finds itself on a new food source starts to divide, with one cell forming two new 'daughter' cells. Each daughter cell can then divide, with the bacterial population growing exponentially and, in many cases, rapidly. Under ideal conditions *E. coli* can divide every 20 minutes and many other bacteria are not far behind. Those bacteria that are most successful at colonising the space will have the greatest numbers and also the best chance of being transferred to new resources. This might be by producing spores (in those species that can do this) or by some other transmission route including, in some cases, by becoming numerous enough to colonise an animal like us and being spread in our faeces or other effluvia. It is divide and conquer, albeit not in the sense that Philip II of Macedon intended.

To prevent other microbes from having the same idea (because, let's be honest, it's a good one), chemical warfare evolved. Those bacteria that can produce chemicals capable of retarding the growth of competitors will prosper, leaving other bacterial dynasties unable to get started. Chemicals that have evolved naturally in microorganisms such as bacteria and fungi to kill other microorganisms have the potential to be used by us to kill bacteria, including those that cause disease. Thus, we enter the world of antibiotics.

There is a reasonable diversity of such compounds already in use, but we are probably only scratching the surface of the Petri-dish pharmacy, since most bacteria haven't been cultured, let alone tested for antibiotic potential. Whether they have broad-spectrum (affecting a wide range of targets) or narrow-spectrum (only affecting specific types) action, whether they are cell-wall attackers, membrane smashers, protein-synthesis saboteurs or enzyme-inhibiting special forces, antibiotic substances are of immense use to us in the fight against pathogenic bacteria. It is important to remember as you read the passages that follow, in which antibiotic resistance and the danger of antibiotic over-prescription are discussed, that antibiotics have saved the lives of countless millions of people. They are wonderful tools in the march of medicine, but like all tools they can be misused and have unintended consequences. An axe is a great tool for cutting down trees, but if you start sharpening your pencil with one then you are going to be donating your gloves to a charity shop pretty quickly.

Thanks to the wonder of synthetic chemistry, we can manufacture antibiotics on a grand scale. Since many can be administered orally they can also be taken on a grand scale, and not just by us. Agricultural livestock can be dosed up with antibiotics even if they aren't displaying any symptoms of illness. This *prophylactic dosing* is used to prevent disease and enhance growth and therefore profit. Of course antibiotics can also be administered if animals display symptoms of gastrointestinal bacterial infection, which can spread rapidly in the relatively close quarters of even the most welfare-conscious farm.

Prophylactic dosing certainly occurs in livestock farming, although the practice has been curtailed since governments have moved to ban the veterinary use of some antibiotics and regulate more heavily the use of others. In 2006, for example, the EU banned the use of whatever antibiotics used to promote growth in farm animals it hadn't already banned.[3] In 2012 the US FDA promoted a more 'judicious' use of certain critical antibiotics used for treating humans in the treatment of animals than had previously been the case. This voluntary initiative aimed at veterinarians, farmers and animal producers especially discouraged the 'production' use of antibiotics to enhance growth.[4] Why the panic? It all comes down to a problem that is rarely out of the news: antibiotic resistance.

Bacteria – always one step ahead

If you are ever faced with someone proclaiming that 'evolution hasn't been proved', then you could perhaps consider acquainting them with one of the truly 'big' problems of the modern world: the evolution of bacteria that are resistant to antibiotics. It's such a big problem that the British Prime Minister David Cameron announced in the summer of 2014 that the world could be 'cast back into the dark ages of medicine' unless we tackled it.[5] It wasn't political posturing (well, it was, but wasn't *just* political posturing), and neither was it especially metaphorical or exaggerated. Mr Cameron's doom-laden warning was in response to a World Health Organization (WHO) report published in April of the same year.[6]

WHO is not given to hyperbole or sounds bites, so when it states that 'A post-antibiotic era – in which common infections and minor injuries can kill – far from being an apocalyptic fantasy, is instead a very real possibility for the 21st century' it feels as if we should be worried. Without antibiotics we are left more or less defenceless in the face of pathogenic bacteria and a great many people will die who, previously, would almost certainly have lived.

Antibiotic resistance – the current picture

Some key findings from the World Health Organization's 2014 report[7] (for the purposes of administration, WHO divides its member states into six regions, which correspond roughly but not exactly to the world's continents):

Resistance to commonly used antibiotics exceeds 50% for the following unwelcome bacteria:

- *Escherichia coli* (virulent strains can cause urinary tract infection (UTI), gastroenteritis and bloodstream infection) in five out of the six WHO regions
- *Klebsiella pneumoniae* (pneumonia, bloodstream infection, UTI) all six WHO regions
- *Staphylococcus aureus* (wound infection, bloodstream infection) five regions

And 25% for:

- *Streptococcus pneumonia* (pneumonia, meningitis, otitis) six regions
- Non-typhoidal *Salmonella* (food-borne diarrhoea, bloodstream infection) three regions
- *Shigella* (bacterial dysentery) two regions
- *Neisseria gonorrhea* (gonorrhoea) three regions

Too important to leave to medics

It's easy to think of antibiotic resistance as a medical issue, but fundamentally it is far too important to leave to medics. Antibiotic resistance is a biological and ecological issue and at its heart is the ultimate unifying idea in modern biology: evolution by natural selection.

To understand how antibiotic resistance works, let's meet a bacterium that has become well known for it, *Staphylococcus aureus*, or more specifically those strains that are known as *MRSA* – the methicillin-resistant *Staphylococcus aureus*. MRSA (sometimes pronounced Mersa, especially in the US) has really caught on in the media and has become a virtual by-word for antibiotic resistance in general. It's a suitably scientific-sounding name for a complex issue, but the problem is that the 'M' and 'SA' in MRSA make the problem look far simpler than it is. They make it seem as if we are dealing with one bacterium that has become resistant to one antibiotic, but this is emphatically not the case. As WHO makes clear:

> . . . resistance to common bacteria has reached alarming
> levels in many parts of the world and . . . in some settings,
> few, if any, of the available treatments options remain
> effective for common infections.

Alarming is one word. Terrifying is another.

Having said that the problem is far greater than just MRSA, given how commonly this 'superbug' crops up in both hospitals and newspapers it is a good case study for how resistance works, how it evolved and how it spreads. But before we embark on some evolutionary science it would be useful to get to know *Staphylococcus aureus* a little better.

Staphylococcus aureus is a spherical bacterium and individual cells cluster together in a way that makes them look like microscopic bunches of grapes. This clustering gives the bacterium the first part of its name: *staphyle* is the Greek word for a bunch of grapes. *Coccus* is from the Greek *kokkos*, meaning granule. Combined, these words give us *Staphylococcus*, which is the name of the genus. It is also a fine example of why scientists refer to the fancy italicised names of organisms as scientific names rather than 'Latin' names. A great many scientific names are Greek, cod-Latin, Latinised names of people or a combination of different origins. A genus is a closely related group of species and in this case the species name *aureus* actually does come from Latin, for golden. When *S. aureus* is cultured on a Petri dish the resulting bacterial colony that spreads across the surface is yellow, hence the name, and this colour distinguishes it from *S. epidermidis*, which is white (for which reason it was initially known as *S. albus*, like albumen, or egg white).

There are more than 20 species of *Staphylococcus*, but *S. aureus* and *S. epidermidis* are the only two that have significant interactions with humans. As with other bacteria, a number of strains have been identified, some of which, as we know, have become resistant to certain antibiotics. *Staphylococcus epidermidis*, as its species name might suggest, is associated with the epidermis, or skin, while *S. aureus* mainly colonises the nasal passages, though it can also be found on the skin, in the mouth and in our gut.

Both species can be pathogenic (cause disease) but *S. aureus* infection is more common and better understood. Infections are characterised by pus. Medically they are termed suppurative infections, although we tend to know them by gloriously old-fashioned terms like pimples, boils, styes, abscesses, carbuncles and furuncles. Such infections, though unpleasant, are medically superficial. *Staphylococcus aureus*, however, can cause more serious problems, including gastroenteritis and potentially fatal toxic-shock syndrome, bacterial pneumonia and sepsis (whole-body inflammation caused by bacterial infection). It's a major source of '*nosocomial infections*', medical jargon for infections acquired in a healthcare setting. Surgical wounds and medical devices that enter the body, such as a cannula in place in a vein and used for drawing off blood or administering drugs, often provide the infection site. Devices that enter our blood system potentially allow *S. aureus* access to the heart, where it can lead to infective endocarditis or inflammation of the inner heart, including the all-important heart valves. *Staphylococcus aureus* is a leading cause of infective endocarditis in otherwise heart-healthy people and medical interventions like cannulae are its main accomplices. It's the potentially fatal aspects of *S. aureus* infection that make hospitals so keen on hand hygiene.[8]

Given the potentially terrible consequences of *S. aureus* infection, it may surprise you to learn that you have a good chance of having it about your person right now. The best places to look for it are the anterior nares, aka the bits of the nostrils that

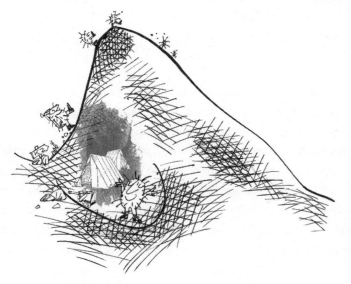

you can poke a finger into. It is here that S. aureus feels most at home, but it is also from here that it can colonise other parts of the body. Studies have shown that if you apply antibiotics and other antibacterial treatments nasally you can actually eradicate S. aureus from the rest of the body, so the bacterium seems to be treating the nose rather like a luxury base camp, with forays out to more remote regions that can be curtailed by making base camp a little less cushy.

Are you a carrier?

People split into three 'patterns of carriage' when it comes to Staphylococcus aureus:

- About 20% of people are 'persistent carriers'. They almost always carry S. aureus and it is present consistently as a particular strain.

- 60% of us are 'intermittent carriers', harbouring S. aureus occasionally with no consistent pattern of which strains we have as our nasal guests.

- 20% are 'non-carriers' and almost never carry S. aureus.[9]

Even among persistent carriers, S. aureus doesn't generally cause many problems. Such a situation is known as *asymptomatic colonisation* rather than infection and, even when it does get a little more serious, most of the pathogenic manifestations of its presence are comparatively minor things like pimples and boils. Serious infections are rare and require bacteria to break through the protective barrier of the skin. Carriage pattern changes with age, with children more likely to be persistent carriers than adults. Many of us will change our carriage pattern between the ages of 10 and 20 and it is interesting that persistent carriers seem to be protected against strains other than the one they are carrying. However, if the carrier is treated with antibiotics, other strains can invade.

Fleming and his mouldy Petri dishes

The fact that we can kill *S. aureus* with antibiotics shouldn't come as any great surprise. For many years we were quite happily treating it with penicillin, for example. It was actually *S. aureus* that Alexander Fleming was culturing when he noticed the adverse effect that the mould *Penicillium notatum* (from which we get the name penicillin) had on it. However, through the 1940s and 1950s researchers started to realise that strains of *S. aureus* isolated in hospitals were developing resistance to the action of penicillin. These strains produced an enzyme called penicillinase that works by breaking down a molecular structure found in penicillin called a beta-lactam. This is a ring of four carbon atoms that lies at the core of the penicillin molecule and is responsible for its antibacterial properties by stopping bacteria of many species building a cell wall, a structure that is essential for bacteria to function.[10] Rare at first, the prevalence of penicillinase-producing strains of *S. aureus* in hospitals began to rise.

This rise in resistance was associated with the end of the second World War and the sudden increase in the availability and use of penicillin for the civilian population. Within a few years virtually all hospital strains of *S. aureus* were resistant to penicillin, although strains found in the 'community' (i.e. not associated with hospitals) remained susceptible and penicillin continued to be used well in the 1970s to treat *S. aureus* infections.[11] The reason why hospital strains of S. *aureus* so quickly and so completely developed resistance is simple mathematics, also known as evolution by natural selection.

Resistance – why maths are against us

Imagine collecting together a whole horde of S. *aureus* on a Petri dish or indeed within a hospital on a population of patients. Just as there is considerable variation within humans, there is variation within bacteria and much of that bacterial variation is genetic and can be passed on to offspring bacteria. Bacterial variation isn't so much about physical appearance (although it could be) as it is about biochemical and metabolic processes, making some better at breaking down or building up certain molecules than others. Some of the bacteria may carry mutations in their DNA, which are mostly small differences in the 'rungs' of the 'ladder' of DNA that lead to a different genetic code. They come about because DNA sometimes needs to be copied and the copying process is not always 100% accurate, introducing rare but sometimes significant errors. Mutations can also be 'forced' by exposing cells to 'mutagens', like UV light, x-rays and certain chemicals.

A different code in the DNA leads to changes in the sequence of amino acids that make up proteins (remember these from Chapter Two?). Such changes more often than not lead to a protein that doesn't perform as well. This is because a different amino acid sequence means that the protein's final shape, so critical to its function, is wrong. For this reason most mutations are harmful, although some are more or less neutral, with the new protein shape being a bit different but not enough to cause any real problems. Alternatively, some individuals will carry certain genes or variants of genes that allow them to do something really beneficial. Sometimes that benefit is only slight, but if the environment changes it can suddenly become huge.

Any *S. aureus* that could produce penicillinase before the 1940s, before hospitals were awash with penicillin, was well placed if it found itself in competition with *Penicillium*, but in the grand scheme of things this type of encounter might be quite rare. As long as the cost of having those genes is small, though, and the chance of encountering an environment where the trait is useful is high enough, then those genes will continue to swill around the population, albeit at a fairly low frequency. However, after penicillin begins to be used widely, those strains that can produce penicillinase suddenly have an enormous competitive advantage over those that don't. The environment has changed drastically and now the encounter rate with penicillin has gone from very low to, in hospitals, virtually unavoidable.

Selective survival is the key

In this new antibiotic-flooded environment, those strains that lack the genes to survive it are at an enormous disadvantage. They die and fail to leave offspring bacteria, while those individuals that can deal with penicillin have the world to themselves. Very rapidly those genes that confer a selective advantage on their bearer increase in frequency until they have, as evolutionary biologists would say, spread to fixation. In a world of penicillin, only the penicillinase-producers survive.

Outside of hospitals, where the environment isn't awash with penicillin, strains that do not carry those beneficial strains can compete on a level playing field and the penicillinase-producers are not able to dominate. Thus two groups of bacteria develop. One group, in hospitals, becomes resistant, while those outside, in the 'community', have far less resistance.

Natural selection is the process by which certain genes, and the bearers of those genes, find themselves at an advantage in a certain environment and prosper, creating offspring with those same genes, who similarly find themselves prospering. Evolution is the resulting change in gene frequency (in this case an increase in penicillinase genes). In bacteria, this process is enhanced by a feature that makes them particularly good at evolving quickly.

Bacteria USB drives

A bacterium's genetic code, the sequence of DNA that, when properly 'read' by the cell's machinery, leads to the production of proteins and to the functioning of the cell, partly exists within the bacterial cell as a circular molecule of DNA called a chromosome. This chromosome sits inside the cell and, unlike human chromosomes, is not enclosed inside a nucleus. If we visualise DNA as a spiralling ladder, then the rungs of that ladder form when so-called base pairs connect with each other across the 'gap'. There are four types of base in DNA and the sequence of these along the DNA molecule is the genetic code. The bacterial genome, though, is not limited to this chromosome. That would be far too simple.

As well as their chromosome, bacteria have 'extra' DNA lurking inside their cells in the form of *plasmids*. Plasmids are small circular DNA molecules that encode for genes that exist entirely separately from the chromosomal DNA. Sometimes there can be hundreds or even thousands of identical copies of these plasmids in a single cell. The useful features that the genes on these plasmids code for include resistance gene.[12]

A helpful analogy for this system is that the chromosomal genome is rather like the hard drive of your computer: full of essential stuff for driving the system, but fixed inside your computer. Plasmids are like a USB drive: small, and not necessarily essential to the working of the system, but very useful nonetheless. An especially handy feature of USB drives is that they can readily be used to transfer information between computers. Likewise, plasmids, and other components of the genome, can be transferred between bacterial cells, including those of entirely different species.

Getting horizontal

The transfer of genes from parents to offspring as a consequence of reproduction is called vertical gene transfer, because those genes go 'down' though the generations. Horizontal gene transfer is the transfer of genes between individuals by any other means. It happens to some extent in eukaryotes, those organisms with a proper nucleus in their large and well-structured cells. To see horizontal gene transfer on a grand scale, though, you need to look at the prokaryotes, in other words bacteria.

We have already encountered some horizontal gene transfer back on the toilet, with the Shiga toxin-producing E. coli strain. In this case genes were probably transferred from Shigella bacteria to E. coli via a bacteriophage, a type of virus that infects bacteria. Bacteriophages, remember, inject their DNA directly into bacterial cells and effectively hijack the molecular machinery of the cell to make new bacteriophages. The manufacture of these new viruses involves copying bacteriophage DNA and this process is not always especially faithful. Some bacteriophage DNA can end up in the bacterial chromosome and the new bacteriophages can end up with pieces of bacterial DNA packaged up inside. The transfer of genes between bacteria via a virus is called transduction and it occurs because of this less-than-perfect copying of DNA and manufacture of bacteriophages.

Unpicking the role of bacteriophages in transferring resistance genes between bacterial strains and bacterial species is still a work in progress, but recent research has clearly shown that bacteriophages 'out there' in the environment do indeed contain genes for antibiotic resistance. The 'out there' that was tested in that study included urban sewage and river water, so these genes are swilling around in the everyday, ordinary environment. But how do they get there?

The passage of genes from bacteria to the wider environment is not a difficult route to fathom. Hospital strains of bacteria that evolve resistance to certain antibiotics could get infected by bacteriophages and some of those phages might end up with resistance genes. Once flushed out into the river system, these phages might infect 'community' bacteria and they could then increase the level of resistance among those strains, even if the community bacteria are not currently being selected for resistance. The transduction route is very real and of increasing interest, but a far greater risk comes from other forms of horizontal gene transfer, notably a one-way transfer called conjugation.

Bacterial special cuddles

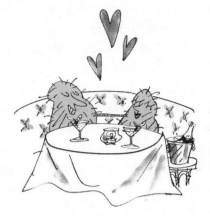

Conjugation is the bacterial equivalent of Mummy and Daddy having a special cuddle. It's just that in this case it's over pretty quickly and involves some very tiny structures. Actually, some might argue it's not that different from regular sex, but the really big difference is that bacterial 'sex' doesn't involve bringing together chromosomal DNA but instead focuses on transferring plasmids. Since antibiotic resistance genes are found on plasmids, conjugation is a very direct and rapid mechanism to spread such genes around a population.

The transfer is, at least conceptually, very simple. One cell acts as the donor cell. Sometimes this cell is referred to as the 'male', but this reference is not especially useful or biologically sound. Males are the sex that produces the smallest sex cells (sperm being much smaller than eggs) and bacteria have enough terminology, jargon, analogy and metaphor without introducing additional confusion into the mix. They don't produce sperm or eggs; the donor is simply the cell that is going to donate a plasmid to another cell, called the recipient.

Many bacteria can produce hair-like appendages on their

external surfaces known as pili, singular *pilus*, which, like the pile of your carpet, comes from the Latin for hair. Pili are made from fibrous proteins and by now you may have got the hang of how proteins are named enough to guess, correctly, that these proteins are called pilins.

Pili have different functions. Type IV pili, for example, are used like molecular grappling hooks, gripping on to a surface and contracting to pull the bacteria closer to that surface. Shorter pili called fimbriae are used to anchor the bacterium to surfaces, which include biological surfaces like our cells and tissues. Fimbriae are essential to colonisation and for the formation of a biofilm and consequently these adhesive appendages are also essential to establishing infections. These pili are very useful for everyday work, but when it comes to bacterial romance the type of pilus with which we need to concern ourselves is unsurprisingly and helpfully called the conjugation pilus.

Not all bacterial cells can produce conjugation pili. The ability to produce the special pilus that allows the transfer of plasmids is itself conferred by the possession of a plasmid termed the F plasmid, with the F standing for fertility. There can be only one copy of the F plasmid in any given cell. Cells that possess a copy of this plasmid are called F-positive or F^+ and can act as donors, whereas cells that lack a copy are called F-negative (F^-) and act as recipients. So far so straightforward ...

A particular chunk of the F plasmid, called *tra*, has DNA that codes for a number of genes involved in the conjugation process, including the pilin gene that codes for the proteins that build the conjugation pilus. The end of the pilus needs to attach to the recipient cell and this attachment is via a protein also coded for by genes in this cluster. And you thought human sex was complicated?

Once the conjugation pilus attaches to the recipient cell, the cells are dragged together and a channel between them is opened by fusing the cell membranes. Once fused, genetic material, like plasmids, can pass between the two cells. It's a very efficient and effective method of transferring useful genes, including antibiotic-resistance genes encoded on plasmids, through populations of bacteria.[13]

Animal resistance

Natural selection, especially in hospitals, for bacteria that can resist the action of antibiotics is also occurring in bacteria that are present in livestock. The widespread use of antibiotics in livestock farming, especially prophylactic dosing of animals to increase growth and productivity, has the same effect on bacterial populations there and, as with hospitals, the same possibility of resistance genes escaping from the 'controlled' reservoir of food-chain animals and into the environment exists. Whether this is actually a danger to human health is open to debate, however, despite the restrictions on antibiotic use in animals put in place by the EU and the FDA. One review, published in 2004, suggested that the 'actual danger seems small' and that 'most of the resistance problem in humans has arisen from human use'.[14] This position still has supporters, while other scientists argue that bans are necessary and can be implemented without harming animal health.[15] This last issue is an important point, of course, because while antibiotics can be used to increase productivity they can also be used to treat sick animals.

Restricting the use of certain antibiotics in livestock against a background of uncertainty as to the true nature of the risk is an example of the 'precautionary principle' in action. We're not totally sure that there is a genuine risk, but there is certainly a theoretical risk and so, some say, it is better to be safe than sorry. Such an approach is not always popular with those scientists who support evidence-based approaches. For example, in the 2004 review mentioned above, the application of the 'precautionary principle' is branded 'non-scientific'. Furthermore, the authors state: 'The banning of the use of growth promoting antibiotics has not been claimed even by its most ardent supporters to have had any detected beneficial effect on human health – and it might even have adverse effects.'

However, evidence has been accumulating and the uncertainty is becoming less and less as research continues. According to some scientists in this field: 'The substantial and expanding volume of evidence reporting animal-to-human spread of resistant bacteria, including that arising from use of NTAs [*non-therapeutic antimicrobials, in other words adding antibiotics to feed to encourage growth*], supports eliminating NTA use in order to reduce the growing environmental load of resistance genes.'[16] Meanwhile, of course, we continue to demand cheaper meat from animals kept in better conditions while expecting any little niggle or infection in our own bodies to be treated immediately and effectively with antibiotics that work. The words 'cake', 'having' and 'eat it' spring to mind . . .

The future

The Darwinian couplet of natural selection and evolution, together with the intriguing methods of gene transfer that have evolved in bacteria and that allow bacteria to evolve very rapidly, have led us to the position in which we now find ourselves. The contribution of each factor and the precise detail of the mechanisms by which resistance is conferred and passed on are in some cases still being worked out, but it is important not to lose the wood for the trees. The bigger picture is startlingly clear and elegantly summed up in the 2014 'Antimicrobial Resistance: Global Report of Surveillance', published by WHO. It's worth re-reading that quote I used at the start: 'A post-antibiotic era – in which common infections and minor injuries can kill – far from being an apocalyptic fantasy, is instead a very real possibility for the 21st century'.

Against all this doom and gloom, there is some hope. We can be more cautious in our use of antibiotics, of course, including their use in animals, and we can gather better information about resistance globally, but we can also tackle things in a more positive manner. If we can develop new antibiotics, then we can start afresh with those and use them in a more judicious fashion. They are not easy to come by: the most recent new class of antibiotics was discovered nearly 30 years ago. Partly this is because of the difficulty of culturing many bacterial species (a problem we first met in Chapter One), but a recent breakthrough in culturing is being hailed as a 'game changer' in ending the decades-long drought in antibiotic discovery. The iChip cultures bacteria in tiny holes in a small rectangular 'plate' enclosed by semi-permeable membranes and this method has already yielded a 'very promising' new antibiotic called *teixobactin*. Tests with this substance, obtained from soil bacteria grown using iChip technology, showed that it could clear a potentially fatal dose of MRSA in mice. Human tests are the next step, but even if teixobactin turns out to be the new wonder drug it will be years before it is available therapeutically.[17]

Looking in new and potentially unusual places might be the key to finding new antibiotics. Scientists working in isolated cave systems in New Mexico, US, for example, discovered a potential novel antibiotic by examining the unusual bacteria that live in these remote systems. What was also interesting was that they found the bacteria there were resistant to virtually all the antibiotics we use! This seems puzzling given their isolation, but remember that antibiotic resistance is a natural phenomenon and bacteria can pass the resistance around through the sharing of plasmids.[18]

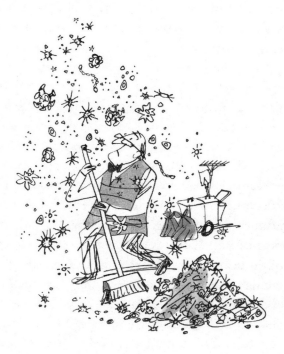

To some extent it feels as if we might always be walking up the 'down' escalator when it comes to bacteria and antibiotics. Perhaps we should be seeking different tools, and indeed some researchers are following alternative routes. Nanotechnology is technology that occurs at a molecular scale, and scientists have recently been considering molecular explosives. Carbon, the black stuff that goes up your chimney and the shiny thing on a diamond engagement ring, can form molecular footballs known as buckyballs. Chemists have simulated adding different molecules to one of these buckyballs to make it explode. So, a buckyball becomes a buckybomb.[19] The simulations of buckybomb explosions show that it could reach 4,000° Celsius in a billionth of a second, and if a bomb could be targeted to attack specific bacteria (and this is theoretically possible), then perhaps they could be blown up?[20] Well, it is one solution, but I wouldn't expect to see a prescription for buckybombs any time soon.

And another thing . . .

Resistance isn't the only issue with antibiotics. As with so many well-intentioned interventions at all scales, there can be considerable collateral damage. The target bacteria may well succumb, but so too may many other bacteria within us that, far from being harmful, are actually beneficial. The resulting fall-out (antibiotic-associated diarrhoea) arises because our well-intentioned intervention disturbs the fascinating and well-balanced community of bacteria living within our gut. It's time to meet them . . .

CHAPTER SIX:

The World Within

In which we become 'internal ecologists' and consider the tremendous diversity and significance of our gut ecosystem, try to imagine 100 trillion and ponder the nature of stability.

Bacteria, as we've seen, are truly remarkable organisms. The relatively vast eukaryotic cell, the sort of cell we find in our bodies, is cluttered in the extreme. The nucleus with its elaborate membranous envelope punctured by protein pores, the fancy *mitochondria* where respiration takes place, the exotically named Golgi apparatus for manufacturing and directing molecules and the seemingly endless endoplasmic reticulum (a membranous network that runs throughout the cell's *cytoplasm*) all look very nice in a biology textbook, and they certainly provide the cell with a dizzying array of functionality, but with size and complexity comes a distinct absence of 'fleetness of foot'.

The stripped-back simplicity and small size of the relatively uncluttered prokaryotic bacterial cell, on the other hand, gives bacteria a tremendous opportunity to exploit niches that larger cells simply cannot enter, including those larger cells themselves. As we have seen, the best-known bacteria, both in the public and scientific worlds, are those that cause diseases in the process of doing exactly that. I have deliberatively focused on these pathogenic bacteria for the first chapters of this book precisely because they are well known. Microbiology is awash with scientific terminology and names that make even the most practised tongues tangle on occasions. Against a background of such linguistic and biological complexity it seems sensible to focus on the familiar, and bacteria like E. *coli*, *Listeria*, *Salmonella* and *Staphylococcus aureus* also provide an excellent framework for getting to grips with some of the more challenging and surprising elements of bacterial biology.

The huge problem with this approach is that it emphasises the harm that bacteria can do, although of course it also echoes the history of bacteria research. From the very beginnings of microbiology it has been the twin quests to understand disease and to provide cures that have tended to force the research agenda. Bacteria from 'out there' do indeed infect us and cause disease and there is no doubt that the wealth of bacteriological research, over the last century in particular, has saved countless millions of lives. But what about the bacteria that live 'in there'? It's time now to continue the journey we started back in Chapter One, delving further into one of the most interesting ecosystems on the planet: ours.

Becoming an internal ecologist

As we have already seen, the bacteria that live in and on our bodies are collectively termed our microbiota and that microbiota includes bacteria that can cause disease under some circumstances. However, as we've also already seen, the connection between bacterial presence and disease is not always clear-cut. For example, healthy people can have thriving communities of potentially pathogenic bacteria like *S. aureus* on their skin or in their nostrils. The nostrils are such a luxurious base camp for *S. aureus* in part because they are moist and warm and we've seen the importance of that microclimatic combination for bacterial growth in other places, too, like the kitchen sponge. The mouth is another warm and moist region and you can feel bacterial growth there with your tongue if you haven't recently brushed your teeth.

With a bit of straightforward management, the bacteria that cause dental plaque and gum disease can be kept in check and any ill effects avoided. Similarly, washing our hands properly, packing our fridges carefully and paying attention to some childishly simple hygiene rules can manage most, if not all, of the problems that bacteria in our bathrooms and kitchens can cause.

When you think about it, a reasonable component of our daily lives is taken up with bacterial management, but in general that management is destructive, seeking to kill those bacteria we believe may cause us harm. With a thriving community of bacteria dwelling within us, though, should we be taking a more benevolent approach to our internal passengers? Should we, in fact, be switching away from pest control, treating bacteria simply as a problem to be killed, and moving towards husbandry, nurturing beneficial bacteria and controlling our internal bacterial communities for maximum health? This approach to medicine is the subject of a later chapter, but for now we need to get to grips with the scale and complexity of our internal world before, inevitably perhaps, looking at what happens when things go wrong.

Awesome abundance . . .

Although many of our surfaces, crannies and orifices provide food and shelter to bacteria, it is our gut that plays host to the highest number and density. Just how many bacterial cells are present in any individual's gut is inevitably an estimate and will be affected by their current health, recent history and physical size. Many estimates seem to level out at around the 100 trillion mark. Although such suspiciously 'round' numbers are best approached with a healthy dose of scepticism, this ball-park figure seems to be widely accepted. Actually the problem with this number is not its roundness but the fact that it is, with the best will in the world, astonishingly meaningless. To give you an idea, here it is written out

Trying to imagine 100 trillion

Consider a regular-sized matchbox. The sort of thing you'd light a cigarette with, not one of those middle-class big boxes with long matches for lighting your wood burner. Such a box is around 4cm long, 2.5cm wide and 1.5cm deep.

If you put 100 trillion of them end to end you'd end up with a line of matchboxes four billion kilometres long.

As a number, that is just as meaningless as the number it's trying to illustrate (which is generally the problem with these big-number analogies), although the boxes would stretch *almost to Neptune*, which feels like trivia knowledge that might one day come in useful.

What about volume? A matchbox has a volume of 15 cubic centimetres and the Great Pyramid of Giza has a volume of about 2.6 million cubic metres.

A cubic metre is a million cubic centimetres, so each cubic metre swallows 66,666.6 recurring matchboxes (with added three-dimensional significance, perhaps, for devil-worshippers), and that means that our 100 trillion matchboxes would have a total volume of 1.5 billion cubic metres.

in full, and remember that in this context a trillion is a thousand billion, and a billion is a thousand million: 100,000,000,000,000. Take a good long look at it and then try to work out what that many marbles, or anything else you care to mention, would look like. Any ideas? Me neither, so I've done a bit of maths to try to put it into context (see box). As I think you'll see, I've failed.

Distressingly, that equates to about 577 Great Pyramids which, although closer to a number I can imagine, is still firmly in the realm of the meaningless!

Taken overall, our microbiota greatly outnumbers our own cells. The cell count of a human body is estimated to be about 37,200,000,000,000 or 37.2 trillion, so our gut microbiota alone outnumbers our own cells by at least three times and, when all our microbiota is accounted for, the multiplier is closer to ten.[1] These numbers also give us a way to understand just how small bacterial cells are, since, despite outnumbering the cells of the body in which they reside, our gut microbiota is estimated to weigh just 1–2kg.

. . . Decent diversity

As well as awesome abundance, our gut microbiota has a pretty decent diversity. It can be a difficult number to pin down and, as we saw in Chapter One, the concept of a species is problematic in bacteria. However, in all, it has been estimated that there are between 1,000 and 1,150 prevalent bacterial species with more than 7,000 different identifiable strains. Of course, we don't all have all of these species all of the time. A healthy individual who has not recently taken antibiotics has around 160–200 species dwelling within him or her, although some estimates suggest that each of us may harbour as many as 1,000 'species-level' varieties.[2]

It is generally the case that additional analyses act to increase rather than decrease our knowledge of diversity, and indeed just a few years ago the total species count was often identified as 800.

To give you some numbers with which to compare 1,000 species, there are, according to the International Union for Conservation of Nature (IUCN), 634 species of primate in the entire world. This group includes us and the other apes, all the multitude of monkeys, the weird and wonderful bushbabies, lorises and tarsiers and the many lemurs that inhabit Madagascar. These are animals that attract more TV time, more cinema characters and more press attention than pretty much any other group, yet are of little ecological significance (with the exception of us) and have a diversity that's not dissimilar to the bacterial diversity you might have expelled into the toilet the last time you defecated. That said, it is hard to imagine E. coli singing 'King of the Swingers', with or without some politically incorrect coconut lip-enhancers.

Our gut is a complex ecosystem

Diversity in ecological systems is often driven by what could be termed habitat complexity. This is the wholly intuitive notion that a more complex environment offers more places to live and more means by which to make a living than does a simpler environment. More complex environments therefore offer more 'niches' for organisms to fill. A niche, sometimes thought of as the 'address and profession' of an organism, is an absolutely central concept in our understanding of ecology, or the study of the interactions and patterns that we see in the natural world. Our gut is not a uniform environment, or, to use a term that crops up in the literature in the area, it is not a uniform 'in-vironment'. There are a number of different, discrete subhabitats within the gut with their own prevailing and sometimes problematic physical, chemical and biological conditions offering a wide variety of potential niches to those organisms able to cope. The stomach, for example, is highly acidic, full of protein-digesting enzymes with a regular cycle of emptying and refilling that creates a rhythmic dynamic that puts me in mind of a rock pool. Only instead of being filled with lovely cool, oxygen-rich seawater, it is full of acidic, chewed-up and partly digested food. Or puke, as it is more commonly called.

If you doubt the powerful acidic nature of the stomach environment, by the way, then you would do well to remember the way your teeth felt after you were last sick. That unpleasant feeling of erosion is the action of hydrochloric acid produced by the glands in your stomach lining and you can but admire the ingenuity of species like *Helicobacter pylori* that are able to make such a challenging, hostile environment their own. This bacterium is found in the stomach of around 40–50% of the population, in most cases probably acquired in childhood and remaining inside the stomach or perhaps venturing into the next section of the gut, the duodenum. For those who have it as part of their in-vironment it can cause problems, specifically stomach ulcers. It's not a simple cause and effect, though. As we've already seen, simply being 'infected' doesn't automatically lead to disease and it's only around 10–15% of people harbouring *H. pylori* who will develop ulcers. But it's not all rosy for the 85–90% who don't, because it is generally agreed that infection with *H. pylori* pretty much inevitably leads to gastritis. What is more, about 1% of those infected with *H. pylori* will develop stomach cancer.[3]

Biologists will drink anything

The discovery of the causal link between H. pylori and stomach ulcers led to Barry Marshall and Robin Warren picking up the Nobel Prize for Physiology in 2005. Part of their research process involved Barry drinking a Petri dish full of the bacterium, which rapidly led to the onset of symptoms associated with a stomach ulcer. This also proves (as I have long suspected) that biologists will drink anything.[4]

The clear risks of H. pylori infection, and the fact that it can be eliminated easily from the stomach using antibiotics, suggest perhaps that a 'test and treat' strategy should be applied to all carriers, a strategy supported by those who have become known as 'treaters'. However, some people, who have become known as 'commensalists', argue that H. pylori is not, per se, a pathogen but is better thought of, in most cases, as a commensal. This literally means 'from the same table' and it is an ecological association of two organisms in which one benefits and the other derives neither benefit nor harm. The commensalists argue that eradication of H. pylori in those not displaying disease symptoms worsens gastro-oesophageal reflux and, they say, can induce asthma[5].

In fact, the commensalists seem to go further and suggest that H. pylori is beneficial, which means that both parties are gaining from the association (the bacteria get somewhere moist and warm to live, albeit a little on the acidic side, and we get a reduction in other symptoms). Such a relationship is properly termed a *mutualism*.

The evidence of the benefit of H. pylori is controversial and far from convincing at the moment, but it's worth considering that this bacterium was only discovered in the early 1980s and there's still plenty that we don't know about it and out relationship with it.

What's interesting is that within medicine the notion of seemingly 'obvious' pathogens potentially having a more complex ecological relationship with their host is being taken seriously, explored and debated.

Entering the intestines

From the stomach our food moves through into the duodenum, passing through a tight sphincter – a round 'balloon knot' of muscle that acts as a secure gateway between internal compartments and between inside and outside. Take a look at a cat's backside, or your own, to get a good idea of what sphincters do.

At around 30cm in length, the duodenum is the smallest component of the three sections that make up the small intestine. The other sections are the Scrabble-player's friend's the jejunum and the ileum, and collectively they are around 7m long. The small intestine is all about chemical digestion (breaking down food into its molecular components) and absorption. It is not a real stamping ground for bacteria: overall, there are fewer than 10,000 bacteria per millilitre here. That might sound like a lot, but remember a gram of soil (which is a slightly smaller volume) might contain 40 million. If bacteria do start thriving in there, they can cause a condition known as Small Intestinal Bacterial Overgrowth (SIBO), resulting in, among other symptoms, nausea, constipation, diarrhoea, bloating, abdominal pain, excessive flatulence and steatorrhoea, an unpleasant sticky form of diarrhoea caused by fats not being absorbed properly and ending up in your poo.

Bacterial overgrowth in the small intestine occurs when species like E. coli, Streptococcus, Lactobacillus and Enterococcus increase in number. The causes are multiple and include diseases that result in a slowing down of the transit of material through the bowel, anatomical problems with that part of the bowel (such as diverticula – pockets where bacteria can accumulate – forming in the bowel), problems with the immune system (more of which later) and conditions where bacteria can pass from the bacteria-rich pastures of the large intestine back into the small intestine.

Whatever the cause, too many bacteria in the small intestine result in poor absorption of nutrients and this causes problems. It can lead, eventually and rarely, to malnutrition, but it also means that the input to the next major compartment, the large intestine, is not what it should be. Components of our food that should have been broken down and absorbed end up flowing into the large intestine and this causes the contents to be more concentrated and less watery than they normally are. As you may recall from school science, water passes through a permeable membrane (like the cells in our intestine wall) from regions with more water to regions with less and this process, osmosis, causes water to pass into the large intestine and subsequently produces watery poo. This is a rather nice example of an ecological problem in our gut. Just as changes to one environment can have unexpected knock-on effects somewhere else, the complex relationships and ecosystem balances in our gut can be disturbed and have consequences downstream.

Into the colon

From the small intestine our food passes into the large intestine or colon, which is the final part of our digestive system. It's only about 1.5m long but, with a diameter of around 7.5cm, it's three times wider than the small intestine. Whereas the small intestine was all about breaking down and absorbing nutrients, the large intestine is about clawing back water and packaging what is left into a nice, neat poo. Like the small intestine it is made up of different components, in this case the caecum, the colon (the main component), the rectum and the anal canal. It is the large intestine that contains the bulk of our gut microbiota.

But what do they get up to down there in that great fleshy tube of poo? Well, the first and most obvious point is that they live there, doing all the usual things that living organisms do, including making new bacteria and feeding. We are, remember, nothing more than an environment as far as bacteria are concerned and the large intestine is a particularly favourable one. However, the relationship between us and our gut bacteria is far from a one-way street. Plenty of their activities benefit us, either directly or indirectly.

Firstly, they assist us in digestion. The mouth, stomach and small intestine, with their digestive arsenal of chewing in the mouth, chemical degradation by acid in the stomach and enzyme action throughout, do a pretty fine job of breaking down food into components that can be absorbed and used by our bodies. What they don't do is a complete job.

We have some wonderful enzymes for breaking down proteins, for example, but our ability to break down some carbohydrates, especially the complex branched sugars that are found in fruits and vegetables, are more difficult to digest and we largely lack the molecular tools, the enzymes, to do it. Some bacteria, on the other hand, with their fabulous array of biochemical pathways and metabolic routes, can digest these molecules, in some cases breaking them down into simple sugars like glucose that we can absorb.[6] These bacteria can also digest the complex branched carbohydrates typically found in mucus, which we produce in considerable amounts from our gut wall to ease the passage of material through our intestine.

Glucose as an end-product is great for us because it is readily used by our cells, but most of the digestive work of our gut bacteria involves converting carbohydrates of different persuasions into short-chain fatty acids by a process known as saccharolytic fermentation. This produces relatively small molecules such as acetic acid (the acidic component of vinegar), propionic acid (which is sometimes used as an preservative in animal and human food because it inhibits the growth of some fungi and bacteria) and butyric acid, which is responsible for the distinctive smell of vomit but is also found in dairy products like Parmesan cheese (be sure to note the delicate hint of sick when you next grate some) and butter, the Latin for which is *butyrum*.

These molecules are readily used by different cells in the body. Acetic acid (in the form of a charged ion called acetate) is used by the liver and muscles, as is propionic acid (again, as a charged ion, this time called propionate). Butyrate is used more or less at the point of production by colonocytes, the cells that form the lining of the colon.

Collectively, the digestive activity of our gut microbiota is considerable and it can be investigated by using germfree individuals. We'll be returning to germfree animals, especially mice, at several points in later chapters, so it's worth committing this to memory now. Germfree animals are raised in isolation from the external environment and are entirely free of colonising bacteria, both inside and out: given the ubiquity of bacteria, this process is by no means straightforward. You possibly have a strong opinion on the use of animals in scientific research, but if we step back from any ethical concerns and consider things from a purely investigative perspective, then germfree animals are clearly ideal for exploring the role of different components of the microbiota in health and disease. Experiments undertaken in rats in the 1980s showed that germfree individuals had to consume 30% more calories to maintain body weight than individuals with a normal microbiota, indicating a significant role of gut microbiota in accessing the nutritional value of food. The complex and ultimately still unresolved issue of human microbiota and body weight is a topic for a later chapter, but in case you started to have a brilliant thought back there, I wouldn't go reaching for the antibiotics if you want to shed a few pounds.[7]

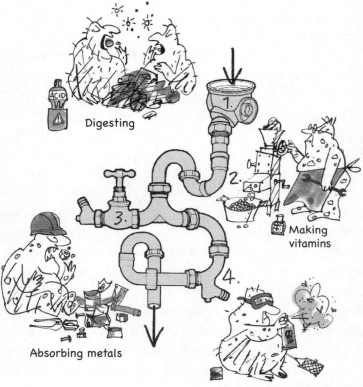

Digesting

Making vitamins

Absorbing metals

Suppressing growth of 'bad' bacteria

Bacteria = farts (the nasty kind)

Saccharolytic fermentation produces hydrogen, carbon dioxide and methane gas that are collectively responsible for about 75% of flatus, or farts. The rest is mostly nitrogen and oxygen that enter our digestive tract when we eat. Together, these gases comprise 99% of flatus and are odourless.

It is the remaining 1%, sulphur-rich compounds such as:

- hydrogen sulphide (the stench of rotten eggs)
- methyl mercaptan (also responsible for bad breath)
- indole
- skatole (derived from the Greek *skato*, meaning dung)

that give your farts that malodorous smell.

Skatole and indole smell of flowers at low concentrations . . . though sadly not at the concentrations present in most farts.

Bacteria are nature's dietary supplement

Secondly, as well as providing a useful service breaking down molecules we love to eat but struggle to digest, our gut bacteria also function as on-board biochemical factories for the production of certain vitamins. These are substances that are vital in very small amounts for our bodies to function but that we cannot make. Our inability to make vitamins means that we have to get them from our food, but poor eating habits (or malnutrition in some cases) can prevent us from acquiring enough to maintain health. Vitamin deficiencies and the diseases they cause, like scurvy (a lack of vitamin C) and rickets (vitamin D) are significant but can be avoided by good nutrition. However, there is another way to acquire vitamins . . .

Right now, in your gut, there are bacteria working away doing what they do, and in some bacteria this includes making vitamins. This is rather useful because it means that, provided we have a healthy gut microbiota, we are able to supplement our diet without resorting to supplements. Certain species of our gut microbiota are able to synthesise and subsequently supply B-group vitamin such as folic acid (B_9 – essential for making and repairing DNA, cell division and growth), biotin (B_7 – required for the synthesis of a number of important molecules in the body) and B_{12} (imporant for our brain, nervous system and blood), as well as vitamin K_2 (necessary for synthesising the proteins needed for blood coagulation).[8] Don't think this is some kind of quick internal fix for a poor diet, though. Bacteria can and do supply some vitamins – and in significant amounts in some cases – but the majority of our vitamin intake comes from the food we eat. Vitamins produced by gut microbiota are also present in potentially useful amounts in faeces and can be acquired by coprophagy which you can observe in some rodents; in other words, by eating faeces. Human faeces also contain some of the vitamins these bacteria have made, but if you want a good source of them I suggest hanging around the stew pot rather than the toilet bowl.

Thirdly, bacteria also do us a favour by making it easier for us to absorb some important metals from our food. We don't often think of ourselves as consumers of metals, but our physiology and anatomy fundamentally rely on metals like calcium (in our skeleton, but also essential if our muscles and nervous system are to work), magnesium (vital for our cells to access the energy bound up in a molecule called ATP) and iron (for making haemoglobin and transporting oxygen). Metals are generally quite reactive and we consume small quantities of them as molecules or as charged ions present in our food. The presence of all those bacterially derived fatty acids in our gut makes it easier for us to absorb these metals.

As if digesting our food, increasing metal absorption and making vitamins weren't enough, our gut bacteria also assist us in suppressing the growth of harmful, pathogenic bacteria by a process that ecologists term 'interspecific competition via competitive exclusion'. Bacteria cause harm by invading cells in our gut lining and, in some cases, subsequently invading other cells in our bodies. Beneficial (or, at the very least, non-harmful) species of bacteria stick to the lining of the intestine and in so doing they use up most of the available space. In other words, they exclude other species by competing for the resources available, the most important of which in this case is living space. This produces a barrier effect, with potentially harmful invading species and ones that are present in normally low numbers struggling to get a pilus-hold on our gut wall. Resident species, selected for their ability to thrive in the gut environment, are often far better at competing for nutrition there and, by fermenting complex carbohydrates into simpler molecules, can produce substances like lactic acid and fatty acids that subtly change the environment to one that suits themselves and hinders competitors. As well as these largely passive actions, resident bacteria can also play dirty, producing bacteriocins. These are protein-based toxins that inhibit the growth of other bacteria, including closely related strains.

Another advantage of gut bacteria, like metal absorption, also stems from the fermentation of carbohydrates to produce fatty acids. The presence of those fatty acids in the gut stimulates the development of the cells lining the intestine, but they also serve to regulate that development, in terms both of the numbers of cells and of cell differentiation: in other words, what sort of cell develops. They also seem to influence the ability of *epithelial cells* to absorb glucose.[9]

It seems to be too good to be true . . .

It's all starting to seem too good to be true and indeed gut bacteria do have some everyday negative effects on our health that are there at a constant level and not related to the more dramatic negative effects caused by the colonisation of pathogenic bacteria. Bacteria in the gut have to eat what we eat. The problem is that bacteria are exceedingly good at consuming pretty much anything we chuck into the system, but most digestive processes produce 'waste'. This might mean components that simply cannot be digested, but it can also be chemical substances that are produced as a by-product of the cunning metabolic sleight-of-hand the bacteria have to perform to process whatever rubbish we've consumed. Diets rich in protein and fat, such as meat-heavy ones, cause our gut bacteria to produce certain nitrogen-rich compounds as a by-product of digesting components of that late-night kebab. These substances, called N-nitroso compounds, are genotoxic, which basically means they can cause serious problems with our DNA. Serious problems with DNA can lead to cancer, in this case colonic cancer. A particular problem seems to be a diet rich in fat and meat but low in dietary fibre: examination of the poo of people consuming such a diet reveals the 'faecal water' (as the researchers term the watery part of the poo) to be high in genotoxic potential.[10]

It's a problem with science that scientists never like to say anything for sure and the link between diet and colon cancer is a good example. The simple fact is that eating a diet rich in meat and fat and low in fibre won't inevitably give you colon cancer. It will certainly increase your risk of getting colon cancer, but the background system of your body is so complex that provoking a simple cause and effect is rarely the right approach. Plenty of heavy smokers don't get lung cancer. People have different genetic backgrounds and different lifestyles, diets and so on and these factors can play an important role in the development of a disease, but are often exceptionally hard to disentangle. In the large intestine, for example, there are bacteria that can induce DNA damage in the presence of heterocyclic amines, nitrogen-rich compounds present in cooked meats, but there are other bacteria that can ingest and detoxify these compounds. The system is rarely, if ever, as simple as we would like it to be and this complexity can make it difficult if not impossible to be 100% certain of anything. Interestingly, the same principle applies in larger ecological situations, where trying to predict the influence of the loss of a species on an ecosystem, or the effects of a new species moving in, is notoriously difficult.[11]

Scientists can be slippery for a reason

Another reason why you can't always pin a scientist down to absolutes is the nature of what scientists consider to be evidence. The scientific method is a pretty simple five-stage process: we see something interesting; we ask questions about it; we formulate some ideas, which we call hypotheses, about what it is, why it might happen and so on; we make some predictions based on those hypotheses; and then we test our ideas in an experiment. Science isn't pub trivia about how far away the sun is or how many bacteria live in our gut; it is an elegant and powerful method for understanding the world. The problems come when we try to work out whether our hypotheses were right.

Some statistics are simply numbers that describe data sets and many of these are pretty familiar. The average or mean (all the data added up and divided by the total number of data points), the total number of data points (typically called N) and measures of the spread of the data (like the standard deviation or the range) are all useful in painting a picture of the data collected, but they don't tell us anything about whether data collected from different treatments (germfree rats versus normal rats) are different (which eats more?) or related in any way. To determine whether that is the case requires us to use inferential statistics, so called because they allow us to infer something about our data rather than simply describe the data.

The output of an inferential statistical test is a value called P, which is the probability of a particular difference or relationship occurring by chance alone. So, perhaps the germfree rats are a little lighter but by chance alone it is quite possible that two samples of rats will have a different mean weight and that the germfree rats will end up the lighter. Such a difference is the consequence of chance differences in sampling rats and nothing to do with their microbiota. What statistics allow us to do is to calculate just how unlucky we'd have to be to observe such a difference or relationship if there was nothing else interesting going on. If that probability, or P value, is low enough (in practice the level is 5% or one in 20) then we say that 'it is highly unlikely that nothing is going on and therefore something interesting is going on and I can support my hypothesis'. So, it is quite possible to get statistical support for a hypothesis on the basis of evidence that could have resulted purely from chance. What is more, hypotheses are never proved; they are only supported, and scientists are therefore never right and are always aware of the probability of being wrong! The problem is that risks and probabilities (and the increasingly used 'confidence interval') are not satisfactory answers to direct questions like 'If I eat this, will I get cancer?' and it's all too easy to think of scientists as being shifty and avoiding straight yes/no answers.[12] Here's the thing, though. If you eat a balanced diet, without a preponderance of meat and fat, you can avoid that increase in risk. It's pretty simple really.

Embrace your diversity: respect your gut!

As well as some clear benefits there is another great reason to embrace and respect your gut bacteria. They are yours. I don't mean this in the trivial sense of them being in your gut. I mean that the bacterial community you harbour in your colon especially is uniquely yours, some say as unique as a fingerprint, although the collection technique required is unlikely to take off in law enforcement.

There are many species of bacteria that all healthy humans share and these core species are dominated by two groups – Bacteroidetes and Firmicutes. Bacteroidetes bacteria are very common and widely distributed bacterial species that are found in soil and water as well as in the guts and skins of many animals. One genus, *Bacteroides*, is the most common species in our gut and is properly regarded as a mutualist, playing a large part in assisting our digestion. The Firmicutes include some familiar names like *Listeria*, *Staphylococcus* and *Clostridium* but they also include a number of less familiar species that are similarly involved in beneficial activities in our gut. People can differ both in the species that are present and in the relative abundance of those species.

Recent examinations of gut microbiota have shown remarkable variations in species diversity and abundance from one gut to another, to the extent that it is possible to identify individuals in the studies based solely on their gut microbiota. This might seem curious, since we all offer similar environments to the bacteria present. However, we differ genetically and that inevitably has subtle effects on our gut as an environment. Also, we are all exposed to different external environments, especially early in life, and we are therefore colonised by different bacteria species and strains. Even identical twins have different gut bacteria, although families do tend to have much more similar bacteria-fingerprints than unrelated individuals.[13]

This pleasing uniqueness might also seem strange given that the positive roles of bacteria in our guts seem to be pretty fixed and rather important to us. The key point here is that, although gut bacterial communities are unique in terms of species diversity and abundance, the overall communities assembled have very similar profiles in terms of the genes that are being expressed. This means that while your gut bacteria are different to mine, both of our gut communities are able to carry out the same functions. Again, there are parallels with bigger ecosystems. Rainforests that look and feel the same on different continents, and have much the same levels of productivity and complexity, possess very different plant and animal species when you examine them at a finer scale.[14]

Another issue in ecology is the idea of resilience. If you disturb a community, does that exact same community develop again, with the same species and the same relative abundances, or is the next community different in terms of species or even in terms of function? The same questions are being asked of the human gut community and the answers at the moment are that the communities we have are pretty stable, and reasonably resilient to change. However, this doesn't mean that species can't change over time, naturally or because of disease or intervention. We'll return to the idea of stability in later chapters.

It's early days in the understanding of our gut as an ecosystem, but this is clearly the direction that biomedical science is taking in order to get to the bottom of bacteria, not just as pathogens but as vital for maintaining health.[15] One aspect of this complex relationship that I've not mentioned yet is the role that bacteria play in our immune system and this role has important links to the best known of all gut problems, the inflammatory bowel diseases . . .

CHAPTER SEVEN

Back to Immunity School

In which we consider how 'Fortress Body' is protected, how bacteria help to teach our immune system friend from foe and how on Earth any of this can be connected to diarrhoea, constipation and inflamed or irritable bowels.

Bacteria, as we have seen, are essential for healthy bowel function. Without them we can neither break down nor digest substantial amounts of the carbohydrates we ingest. What is more, they provide a drip-feed of some vitamins essential for a variety of bodily functions: they increase our ability to absorb metals; they regulate the production and function of cells lining our intestine; and they prevent harmful bacteria from proliferating. In exchange we offer them a relatively safe home, ideal growing conditions and the opportunity to spread to other environments, a distribution greatly enhanced by our generally poor hand hygiene and the capacity of young children to put pretty much anything into their mouths. It's a wonderful relationship that is really only soured when we do something to disturb this otherwise stable community, by consuming potentially pathogenic bacteria (akin to introducing a non-native species to an ecosystem) or nuking everything by taking antibiotics.

However, there is one other thing that we have only recently realised that gut bacteria do for us and that it is absolutely crucial for good health. They help to teach our immune system.

'Fortress Body'

If we think of our bodies as a castle, then the skin is the moat and the walls. It is our first line of defence against the outside world and serious problems can occur if it is breached. Should intruders, such as bacteria, make it through the castle walls, then our immune system is there to deal with the problem.

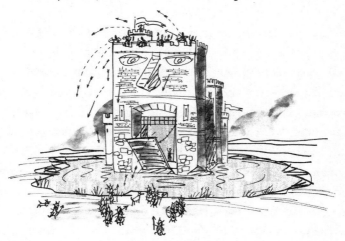

Our immune system is a remarkable network of cells, tissues and organs that work together to attack and destroy invaders. White blood cells, or leukocytes, are one important part of the system. These are made and stored in places like bone marrow and the spleen and they are also housed in 'barracks' at more far-flung sites in the empire of the human body, such as the lymph nodes. These cells circulate using blood vessels and the other great transport system, the lymph vessels. Patrolling around the body, they are constantly on the lookout for potentially problematic invaders.

There are two basic types of white blood cell. *Phagocytes* ingest invading cells and include an important group called the *neutrophils*. Neutrophils are both the most common phagocytes and the cells that target bacteria. If we have a bacterial infection, then the number of neutrophils increases in response to the increasing threat. The second type of cell are the *lymphocytes* and there are two categories of these, B-lymphocytes and T-lymphocytes (also called B- and T-cells), so called because they mature in the thymus, an organ of the immune system located near the heart. T-lymphocytes are also produced and stored in the tonsils, which is handy when you think about keeping the name simple. Both cells start off in the bone marrow, but unlike T-lymphocytes the B-lymphocytes stay there. (The name B-lymphocyte, by the way, comes from an organ in birds that is similar to the thymus in mammals and located near to a bird's backside, or cloaca. This organ has a wonderful name that sounds more like an officer on an ancient Roman cruise ship than an organ of the immune system: the bursa of Fabricius.)

The system is beautifully elegant when it works properly, but it is also very complex. The picture usually painted is one in which invading cells are recognised because of molecules on their cell membrane that differ from the molecules our own cells have. Such recognition factors are termed antigens, and antibodies are produced in response to the detection of these antigens. Antibodies stick to the invader's cell membrane, marking it for subsequent killing by the phagocytes. This basic model of the immune system is sound and many bacteria are indeed killed this way, but there are other mechanisms whereby invading bacteria can be hunted down. First, when some bacteria invade they can be targeted by specific immune proteins called complement proteins. These can recognise antibodies and bind with them, causing further proteins to come and join the party, collectively becoming a membrane attack complex (MAC), a kind of small elite Special Forces protein team that can breach the cell membrane and eventually cause the cell to collapse.

Bacteria are not helpless in this concerted attack against them. Organisms and invading bacteria are in a constant arms race, with natural selection and evolution providing the next measures and counter-measures in an escalating conflict. With their rapid generation time and other genetic tricks like plasmid sharing, bacteria might be expected to have the advantage, and sometimes they do. Some bacteria, like *Salmonella*, can avoid being killed by the cells of the immune system that ingest them and, as we know, can cause serious problems. But, in the arms race of the immune system, these white blood cells have a trick up their sleeve. They can present peptides (chains of amino acids) from the bacteria they have engulfed on their external membranes. These act like molecular flags, signalling to a type of T-lymphocyte called a helper T-cell to come and release a molecule that helps the hapless white blood cell overcome its internal invader.

Second, some of our immunity is present from birth. This innate immunity involves white blood cells exercising the simple but powerful principle of sniffing out invaders and neutralising them. The innate immune system can recognise and deal with certain kinds of infection without any need to learn to distinguish 'good' from 'bad'. This is pretty useful, because any system of learning is time-consuming and, with the high rate of population expansion possible in bacteria, it is as well to have a general strategy to deal with most problems quickly and effectively. However, it doesn't work if we are invaded by something that the system cannot recognise.

Coping with novel invaders

The adaptive immune system, on the other hand, can cope with novel invaders, although there is an inevitable lag period when we are first exposed. The adaptive system, which makes use of B- and T-lymphocytes, can learn to recognise harmful invaders because these invaders do not have 'self' antigens, specific molecular flags, on their membranes. The B-lymphocytes can create antibodies that bind to the invaders and, together with the T-lymphocytes, the cells can mount an attack. What is particularly useful with this system is that it remembers these novel attackers and if they are encountered again the response can be much faster, without the need to re-learn.

At first glance, the immune system might appear to be something of an obstacle for gut bacteria trying to set up home within us. One way or another it would seem that we have the immunity tools to destroy them without too much fuss and bother. It used to be thought that this wasn't any sort of problem for gut bacteria because they were essentially isolated from our immune system. Living as they do in the space and walls of the gut they would only come into contact with the immune system when they breached this protective layer and entered the 'body' properly. You might get into the sewerage system of a castle, but you are only going to cause a problem and be identified by soldiers within when you emerge from a toilet. However, we now know that gut bacteria and the immune system are in rather close and important contact with each other.

Surviving in enemy territory

Microscopic examination of intestines of mice has revealed that gut bacteria live in habitats that put them into intimate association with the immune system. Located deep within crypts in the intestinal wall, bacteria and the immune system can communicate with each other and, as in all relationships, it is communication that is vital in maintaining cordial rapport.

Bacteroides fragilis is found in mice but is also a beneficial member of our gut biota. This bacterium is able to stay in the gut despite having the potential to be recognised by the immune system. Research into how bacteria are able to reside in such a potentially hostile environment has revealed an elegant but complex chain of molecular communication and responses.

The bacterium produces a complex sugar molecule called polysaccharide A or PSA. Complex polysaccharides, molecules that have sugars as their fundamental building blocks, are excellent recognition molecules because they have a dazzling variety of possible structures and these structures have the potential to be recognised by cells. In this case, PSA on the surface of the bacterium is recognised by one type of cell in the adaptive immune system, the regulatory T-cells, or *Treg cells*. Treg cells usually prevent the immune system from reacting to and attacking the body's own cells. They do by this by shutting down some of our immune responses at appropriate points. If we have a problem with this system, then the immune system can no longer distinguish friend from foe and can attack everything, causing an autoimmune response that can lead to diseases like Guillain-Barré syndrome (which we met in Chapter Three), multiple sclerosis and lupus.

The PSA is detected by receptors on the surface of the Treg cells called toll-like receptors. Once the Treg cell's toll-like receptors detect the PSA, the cell is activated to suppress the activity of another type of T-cell, T helper 17 (Th17).[1] To extend the castle analogy a little further, the T helper cell is like an assassin inside the castle and the Treg cell is like a guard. When the 'friend' bacterium appears at the gate, the guard recognises it and tells the assassin to back down and leave it alone.

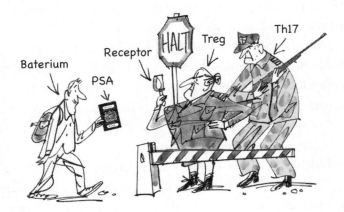

As you can tell, the immune system is a bit more complex than I made out earlier, but it needs to be when you consider the scale and complexity of the problem it has to solve. Without the interference of the Treg cell, the guard at the gate sifting friend from foe, the Th17 cells would normally trigger an inflammatory response and stimulate gut-lining cells to produce antibacterial proteins to deal with the offending invader. By shutting down the Th17 response, the bacterium avoids such an attack. This is a pretty neat solution to the bacterium's problem of staying in the gut, where food and shelter are a given, and to the host's problem of wanting to offer that food and shelter to something that every internal security system wants to destroy.

Normally, triggering toll-like receptors on the surface of Treg cells activates the pathway that results in the elimination of bacteria. The bacterium and host have co-evolved a way that allows the host to keep a tight security system active against harmful bacteria while recognising those that are beneficial. Our adaptive immune system has to learn to identify these bacteria but, once it does, they are free to stay, to the mutual benefit of both parties.

If you remove the PSA molecule from the bacterium, or the PSA receptor from Treg cells, or the Treg cells themselves, then the situation changes rapidly. Without any way to tell the host, 'It's me, please don't kill me', and with no way to stop the ever-active Th17 cells from doing their work, the bacterium is now treated as a harmful invader by the host system, which mounts a robust immune response to deal with it.

Intimate relationships

Our immune system has evolved to respond quickly and effectively in the face of some challenging adversaries, but it seems also to have developed flexibility, which allows us to accept a wide variety of bacteria whose presence can be beneficial. The relationship between our gut and our immune system is really in its infancy as far as scientific research and development go, although the idea that there might be a relationship dates back more than 40 years. Research in this area is ramping up, and more details on the mechanisms and the implications of the relationship will be a significant feature of the next 20 years or more of biomedical research.[2] If I were writing this book in 2035 the basic message, that the relationship we have with bacteria is complex and crucially important, would not change, but I'm confident that the scale of both the importance and complexity would change immensely. It's exciting to think that right now someone is probably working on research that will lead eventually to Nobel Prizes, but it's also sobering that our present understanding, though impressive in many respects, is akin to that of a toddler looking at a blackboard full of astrophysics equations.

The beneficial microbiota and our immune system work together to ensure that beneficial microbes are tolerated, but it is also crucial that an immune response can be mounted against pathogenic bacteria should they make an appearance. Rather like a nightclub doorman, the system needs to strike a balance between letting everyone in and keeping everyone out, but the club owner (which in this analogy is the host's body) needs to make sure there are enough doormen. Sure enough, the relationship between gut bacteria and our immune system doesn't stop at recognition and learning. Remember those Th17 cells that are part of the inflammatory response? Well, it turns out that the production of these cells in the gut wall is closely linked to the presence of certain bacteria in the microbiota of the gut. Indeed, the results suggest that the composition of the microbiota in our gut regulates the balance of Treg and Th17 cells in the intestine wall and that therefore the normal, healthy gut microbiota plays an influential part in the immunity, tolerances and susceptibilities of our gut.[3]

The embers in the fireplace

So, we now know that our microbiota plays an incredibly important role in the development and regulation of our immune system,[4] as well as in its homeostasis, the term biologists use for the process of keeping a biological system stable. This homeostatic function is achieved in part through the relationship between the gut microbiota and the production of Th17 and Treg cells, and one scientific paper provides a pleasing metaphor for it. In a poetic flourish not normally seen in bacteriologists writing scientific papers, the authors liken the host immune system to a house and the beneficial microbiota to the embers in a fireplace. At homeostasis the embers are glowing and providing constant minimal heating for the house, but when an immune response is needed they help to create a powerful flame.[5]

Why does the house sometimes burn down?

At a healthy equilibrium your gut bacteria are vital for your immune system and it seems perfectly reasonable to say that they are, essentially, a *part* of your immune system. But what happens when things go wrong, when the embers flare up and start heating the home in the middle of a summer's day, or burn the house down altogether? Increasingly, research is finding links between a seemingly disconnected set of diseases and our gut bacteria. These include obesity and allergies (covered in Chapters Eight and Nine), but the diseases most commonly linked to gut microbiota and the immune system are the inflammatory bowel diseases of Crohn's disease and ulcerative colitis.

Crohn's disease is a long-term condition that causes inflammation of the lining of the digestive system. It can affect anywhere from the mouth to the anus but it most commonly occurs in the ileum (the last and main section of the small intestine) and the large intestine, sites that also, interestingly enough, harbour the highest abundance and diversity of bacteria. Crohn's disease causes a suite of symptoms that include diarrhoea, abdominal pain, blood and mucus in your poo, weight loss and extreme fatigue. These symptoms can cause damage to the gut that requires surgery to remove or repair. Symptoms can be mild or even disappear completely when the disease is in remission, only to flare up later and cause considerable problems. Living with Crohn's is, by all accounts, miserable and its incidence and prevalence are increasing in the developed world.[6]

It's worth stating clearly that at the time of writing we don't know for sure what causes Crohn's disease. What we do know is that some unknown factor or combination of factors triggers the immune system to produce an inflammatory response in our gut that continues running out of control, provoking the characteristic symptoms of Crohn's. To extend our embers analogy, the sun is shining, the windows are open and the rum coolers are poured, but in the fireplace the glowing coals have flared up and are now burning the curtains.

Although the details are still to be determined, over the past few years a consensus seems to have been reached that combines three different contributory factors into a model for understanding the disease. Those factors are genetics, environmental triggers and a strong role for gut bacteria and while it is tempting to think of them acting together as separate entities, they are to a certain extent intertwined. To understand them we first need to consider our genes.

I have nothing to declare but my gene-ius

It may disturb some people's view of the human world and of themselves to learn this, but a great deal of the 'you-ness' about you is purely genetic. This isn't a manifesto for biological determinism or a denial of free will (although the freedom of much of what we do in our everyday lives is questionable), but a statement of fact. You are a physical, organic being that has developed as a consequence of the genetic information encoded in your DNA. Certainly, some important aspects of you have developed as a consequence of the interplay between this genetic background, your genotype and the environment in which you grew up, but many of the physiological, anatomical and biochemical features of you are hard-wired in your genes and, at the moment, there is not a lot we can do about that. Research into the link between inflammatory bowel disease (IBD) and genotype has revealed that some people have a genetic susceptibility to these problems.

A common trope in media stories reporting links between some feature of human physiology, pathology or behaviour and our genome is the 'gene found for' headline. In reality, complex biological phenomena like behaviour or the immune system are polygenic, meaning they are under the influence of large numbers of genes. Typically 'a gene has been found' is journalistic shorthand for 'a genetic link involving multiple genetic regions has been supported' and in the case of IBD it is very much a simplification, since researchers have found more than 160 genetic regions associated with it. Interestingly, there is a vast amount of overlap genetically between Crohn's disease and ulcerative colitis, strongly indicating that they are indeed closely related diseases with similar biological pathways within the body.

Taken individually, each of the genetic regions with a link to IBD has only a tiny influence on a person's likelihood of developing the disease. Even if the influence of each individual genetic region could be considered together it would not result in a foolproof way of determining whether or not the holder of any particular genetic profile would develop IBD. What this knowledge does provide is information on the many biological pathways that are implicated in IBD and that gives researchers clues as to where to look for further insights.[7]

It is possible to determine which genes are being actively used or 'expressed', in cells and, when the activity of genes in the IBD regions was studied in the many cells that make up the immune system, it was the cells that are involved in the body's first line of defence against bacterial invasion that had the most gene expression. Evidence for a close connection between the immune system and IBD is further provided by a comparative approach in which the IBD-associated regions are compared with other diseases. What this approach revealed was that 70% of the genetic regions associated with IBD are shared with complex diseases like psoriasis and ankylosing spondylitis, the symptoms of which are driven, like IBD, by inflammation. Comparing the genetic regions with genes associated with susceptibility to leprosy and tuberculosis revealed yet more intriguing insights. These diseases are caused by infection with mycobacteria and again there was a strong overlap between the susceptibility genes in these diseases and the genetic regions associated with IBD.

Although the precise details are still being worked out, we do know that the genetic component of IBD is strong. In fact, a family history of IBD is the biggest known risk factor: those with a close relative (parent, sibling) with IBD have about a one in ten chance of developing it themselves, compared to a general incidence of one in 10,000.[8]

The recipe for our immune system is encoded in our DNA and it is clear that in some people it contains a few potentially dangerous typing errors. The recipe can still make a cake that mostly looks, tastes and smells about right but it can also, in certain cases, set the oven on fire and burn down the kitchen. Exactly what triggers the immune system to go rogue is hotly contested. Again, the media like to play a simple tune, so headlines abound blaming diet, cigarette-smoking or stress for triggering the onset of IBD, particularly Crohn's disease. In reality, given a complex genetic background and an equally complex internal environment, it is entirely possible that a range of different triggers may be responsible, and that those triggers may vary from one individual to another. However, while the environmental triggers of IBD are still debated, the strong role that the gut microbiota plays in IBD is becoming very clear.

Postulates and beyond

The traditional medical understanding of diseases that are likely to be caused by microbes is underpinned, at least historically, by what became known as Koch's postulates. Robert Koch was a German physician regarded as the father of the study of bacteria and celebrated for his part in identifying the bacteria that cause tuberculosis, cholera and anthrax. Through his research he developed four criteria for linking a specific microbe to a specific disease. These criteria – or postulates – became the guiding principles in biomedical disease research in the last century. They have been largely superseded by revised principles that include aspects of DNA and gene expression that were unknown to Koch, but nonetheless the logical scheme that Koch's postulates provide remains useful. They state that the microbe must be found in abundance in those suffering from the disease but not in healthy individuals; that it should be able to be isolated and cultured from a diseased individual; that the cultured microbe should cause disease when introduced into a healthy individual; and that the identical microbe should then be able to be isolated and cultured from the newly infected experimental host.

We are still discovering gut bacteria and many of them

cannot yet be cultured, so satisfying Koch's postulates could well be difficult for any candidate causal bacterium of IBD. So far, in fact, no bacterium has been identified as the cause, although it is still possible, given the tremendous amount of 'known unknowns' and the very high likelihood of 'unknown unknowns', that a species of bacteria could be the cause of IBD. Various species have been suggested, including a mycobacterium that causes a similar disease in cattle, a specific strain of *E. coli* and cold-tolerant bacteria such as *Listeria*. Sensible money doesn't appear to be backing this scenario, though, and the connection between our microbiota and IBD seems not to be one of simple 'one bacterium' cause and effect, but instead probably involves the balance of the microbial community as a whole.

This community approach is exemplified by a recent study encompassing more than 650 people. This study showed that Crohn's disease was associated with increased abundance in bacteria, including the Enterobacteriaceae, Pasteurellacaeae, Veillonellaceae and Fusobacteriaceae, and a decreased abundance of Erysipelotrichales, Bacteroidales and Clostridiales. What was also interesting was that antibiotic exposure exaggerated the microbial imbalance that was associated with Crohn's disease: in other words, antibiotics can make it worse, not better. The authors of this study go so far as to suggest that comparing the microbes in the small intestine, the rectum and in poo might offer a chance for easy and early diagnosis.[9]

Blessed are the peacemakers

Having said that the 'one bacterium' smoking gun seems unlikely, there is one bacterium, or more accurately its absence, that has been strongly implicated in Crohn's disease. *Faecalibacterium prausnitzii*, present in abundance in healthy guts, has been found to be very much reduced in the guts of people suffering from Crohn's disease. This species has become known as a peacekeeper bacterium and tests in mice and in test tubes have revealed that, like some other species, *F. prausnitzii* is a powerful anti-inflammatory member of the gut microbiota. These peacekeepers help to maintain a healthy mucus layer on our gut lining, keeping the walls of the castle intact. They also help to soothe the immune system. Dwelling in the mucus lining, they are mostly fermenting dietary fibre that we cannot digest (more of which in Chapter Ten), but if there is none of that about they can also digest sugars in the mucus itself.

From an ecological perspective, what is especially interesting is that peacekeeper bacteria seem to be able to stimulate the production of mucus. We are truly in partnership with these bacteria, supplying them with nutrients through our diet and through mucus production, which encourages other beneficial bacteria to grow, outcompeting the potential foes and preventing them from accessing the cells of the colon. At the same time, some of these species are preventing inflammation and calibrating our immune system.[10] It is a story of ecological subtlety and one that is constantly developing. It is also a story that starts to present some obvious 'ecological' therapies . . .

Anyone for tennis?

Think of your gut bacteria as being like the plants in a lawn. I don't mean a well-tended Wimbledon-like monocultural sward with stripes, I mean more the sort of patch of grass many of us have outside the back door. If we take a look at that 'grass' we'll see that there are actually an impressive number of different species of plants poking their heads through. In addition to several species of grass, we'll likely see clovers, dandelions and daisies, as well as some less familiar plants that we only notice when they flower. What looks, from a distance, to be homogeneous and simple is, up close, a complex biodiverse ecosystem. Unless we are particularly fastidious gardeners, we are more concerned with its usefulness than with its make-up. Can the kids play football on it, can we look at it and feel good, and can the dog go to the toilet on it? The exact species composition doesn't matter as long as the overall community functions as it should. Sometimes, though, something happens to disturb the balance of our lawn. Perhaps the grass starts to die back and dandelions take over. Now, what used to be a welcome little splash of colour becomes a rampaging weed and the lawn is no longer so nice to look at, or to play football on. The species composition has shifted and the resulting community has different properties that are less desirable.

So it is with our gut microbiota and recent work has shown that people suffering from IBD have distinct changes in their gut bacterial community.[11] Some bacteria, the dandelions, increase in abundance, while others, the grasses, decrease, creating a disturbance in the usual healthy balance. 'Good' bacteria, normally tolerated by the immune system, are suddenly targeted by it, while 'bad' bacteria are allowed to flourish. Meanwhile, the immune system is responding to the perceived 'threat' and causing inflammation. On top of direct immune responses, the different bacterial community also changes the biochemical environment of the gut because the proliferating bacteria have different ways of fermenting our undigested and partially digested food.

All paths lead to gut bacteria

We like a neat story when it comes to disease. People get symptoms, we work out what is causing them and we come up with a cure. Uncertainty, especially over diseases that are 'common' (or at least, that we perceive are common) and seem to be increasing in frequency, makes us understandably nervous. It feels as if we are so technologically advanced that we should be able to fix anything. The problem with IBD is that while people continue to get symptoms, and we continue to develop a decent understanding of these symptoms and their implications, a straightforward answer has not yet been found. All paths seem to lead to gut bacteria, but even then the situation is not as simple as we would like, with imbalance at a community level rather than a single 'bad' bacterium seemingly at fault. It is tempting to consider treating IBD with antibiotics, which indeed is a frequent course of action when patients present with mild symptoms. However, even that solution is not always effective because, far from restoring the balance, this approach cluster-bombs the already imbalanced ecosystem and can make the symptoms worse, at least according to some research.[12] What we are left with is a situation where we can't cure IBD because we don't know for sure what causes it. The good news is that we are getting there. The bad news for sufferers is that we are certainly not there yet.

Feeling irritable?

As well as IBD, there is another abbreviation that can cause problems with our guts, IBS or Irritable Bowel Syndrome. Symptomatically it is tempting to think of these conditions as similar. Both cause a painful gut and diarrhoea, for example, but they are actually quite different. IBS is what is sometimes called a functional disorder and is, despite causing much distress, a less serious condition. IBD, remember, can cause such injury to the bowel that only surgery can rectify it, and this is not the case with IBS, where the bowel remains generally intact but doesn't work quite as it should. Consequences of this dysfunction include painful abdominal cramping, bloating, flatus, mucus in your poo, diarrhoea (which is associated with virtually everything, of course) and, conversely, constipation. IBS is a chronic condition but its progression is uneven, with flare-ups and periods of relative calm being a common pattern. It is well established that flare-ups can be caused by stress and also, cue alarm bells, antibiotic usage.[13]

With bacteria proving to be so crucial to IBD, it is perhaps not surprising that they have also been found to have an influence in IBS. If anything, that influence is even more 'ecological' in IBS, with studies exposing hidden connections and complexities within our bodies, connecting a variety of important control systems to our gut bacteria and even affecting our brain and the way we perceive the world. Sufferers of IBS, for example, have increased levels of anxiety and depression and they also have a lower pain threshold than those without IBS.[14] By the way, this pain threshold is measured by the balloon distension test, which is a nice way of saying that someone inflates a balloon in our gut and we tell them how much it hurts. These apparent psychological and pain-related symptoms suggest that changes in the gut can affect far more than how often and how unpleasantly we need to go to the toilet.

Recently, some researchers proposed a model to explain the long-term gut dysfunction associated with IBS. The chain of events is lengthy and involved. In essence, their model suggests that the chain reaction starts with a trigger event, which might be infection, stress or antibiotic usage. This trigger causes dysbiosis, a detrimental imbalance in our bacterial community, in this case in our gut. Detrimental bacteria proliferate at the expense of beneficial species and this causes a change in our physiology, or the way that our bodies work at a fine scale. The dysbiosis linked to IBS causes changes in the way our gut contracts to move digested food through it (gut motility), changes in hormone secretion and changes in the production of mucus by our gut lining. Collectively, these changes alter the chemical and physical habitat of the gut. It is rather like suddenly shading the lawn we met earlier, and turning on the sprinklers. These new conditions select for different species and strains of gut bacteria, which leads to instability in the gut microbiota community.

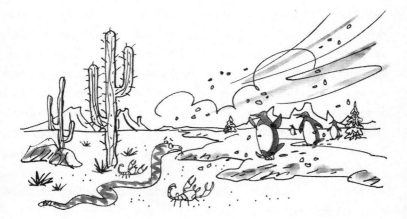

This instability leads to further changes in the habitat of the gut, leading to more changes in microbiota, and thus a self-perpetuating vicious cycle is established, with chronic gut dysfunction and microbiota community instability as the consequences.[15] This model of IBS is not yet fully established, but all the signs are good that the researchers, by combining knowledge gained from a range of animal and human studies and clinical trials, are on the right lines.

Links between gut bacteria and our gut health feel intuitively right. However, with IBS comes insight into a more intriguing and far less intuitive situation. Studies with germfree[16] and normal mice have shown that behaviours associated with anxiety are linked to the bacterial status of the gut and that manipulation of the gut microbiota can alter the behaviour of the animals. Bacteria in the gut have also been shown to affect brain chemistry in mice, causing changes in learning, memory and emotive behaviour. Remarkably, in one study, transplanting gut bacteria from one group of mice into another via a faecal microbiota transplant (FMT, more of which later) resulted in 'transplanting' some of the behavioural characteristics from donor to recipient.[17] Taken together with the observation of reduced pain thresholds and increased anxiety in human IBS sufferers, this raises a whole host of interesting research questions as to how our gut bacteria might be affecting us. It seems that even as we enter the brave new bacterial world, understanding that gut bacteria are more complex than we thought, we already have to pop through a wormhole into another universe of understanding that goes far beyond the childish 'bacteria in our tummies can cause problems in our tummies' understanding. Bacteria may change the way we think, the way we act and the way we feel. We'll explore the gut–mind connection more in Chapter Nine.

It's a complex world in there

IBD teaches us a valuable lesson about our gut community. A 'Koch's postulate', one-disease-one-bacterium approach doesn't seem to be the right one to take, although people sought the cause of peptic ulcers for a long time before Barry Marshall took on Koch's postulates and *Helicobacter pylori* in one unpleasant drink. It is still possible that a single bacterium could be responsible, but the evidence is increasingly pointing towards IBD being the consequence of an ecological disturbance of our gut bacteria, perhaps triggered by smoking, stress or some other factor and underlain by a complex genetic susceptibility. The complexity of interactions in the world with which we are familiar, the 'big' world with mammals, birds and insects, means that we often struggle to predict the effect of new species on even simple ecosystems that we have studied for more than a century. The study of the complex ecosystem of our gut is really just beginning, so it is perhaps not surprising that gut ecologists are still catching up. We can, though, already see a distinct shift in the way that the medical world is approaching this aspect of health. What if, as well as fixing gut ecosystems that have gone haywire, we 'weed and feed' our internal lawn to keep it healthy, or transplant new species to develop a favourable equilibrium? Before we talk about gut husbandry and poo-eating, though, we need to consider some of the other surprising connections and influences our internal passengers are having on our health.

CHAPTER EIGHT

It's not my Diet, Doctor, it's my Bacteria

In which we consider the connections between bacteria and obesity, the dolphin of consensus and the wisdom of Benjamin Franklin. And we absolutely don't blame bacteria for our being fat.

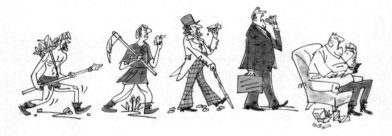

The idea that our gut microbiota could have far-reaching implications for digestive health doesn't seem like a great intellectual stretch. OK, we still don't know the exact causes of IBD or IBS, but we are starting to appreciate that it's a complex picture. It is also clear that bacteria are firmly in the sights of those chasing down first the cause of and then the cure for these conditions, especially IBD. Recently, bacteria have been implicated in other health issues that initially seem less likely to have a bacterial angle: obesity and the rise of allergies. However, armed with knowledge of our in-vironment and fortified with an ecological viewpoint of our inner world, these relationships suddenly do not seem so far-fetched.

We'll cover allergies in the next chapter but for now let's start with the biggest problem, in every sense. Obesity is just medical jargon for having a BMI (body mass index: your weight in kilograms divided by your height in metres squared) of greater than 30, but for once let's be straightforward and honest about this condition. Let's call it what it is: being fat.

From lean, fast and strong to fat, slow and weak

Getting fat, and staying that way, is fundamentally about eating too much or, more accurately, ingesting more energy than you expend. We have a wonderfully evolved physiology, adapted to a lifetime of feast and famine, and when we feast on more than we need, our body, ever cautious of future famine, stores the surplus in the form of fat. Fat is our on-board energy storage technology and a very effective one it must have been for our ancestors, actively eking out an existence from kill to kill via whatever berries, nuts and roots they could hunt and gather. The modern lifestyle is very different. We are essentially sedentary and, what is worse, our sedentary modern selves are surrounded by calorie-dense food, loaded with yummy fats and sugars. The inevitable consequence is that we end up consuming more than we need, and our wonderfully adapted physiology works against us by stashing away the surplus under our skin for a future famine that will never materialise. Humans, once lean, fast and strong, have become, purely through lifestyle choices, fat, slow and weak.

It is now commonplace to refer to obesity as an epidemic and it is worthwhile chewing over some of the latest facts and figures from the World Health Organization so that the scale of the problem is fully appreciated (Fact Sheet No. 311, if you fancy something to read over your mid-morning doughnut).[1]

Worldwide obesity has nearly doubled since 1980 and, quite shamefully, 65% of the world's population now lives in countries where more people will die from eating too much than from eating too little. Thirty-five per cent of those over 20 are overweight; 11% are medically obese; and more than 40 million children under the age of five were overweight in 2011. Childhood obesity is a particular concern and some argue that it is a particularly damaging form of abuse, which through the perpetuation of harmful eating habits and a culture of poor nutrition is likely to persist across generations.

Don't blame your bacteria!

Obesity is an entirely preventable medical condition and nothing I am going to say about the role of bacteria changes this simple fact. You are not fat because you have the 'wrong' bacteria. You are fat because you have the wrong diet for you and your in-vironment. I guess what I am saying is don't treat gut bacteria like the new 'slow metabolism' or 'bad genes' and don't blame them if you find that your clothes are shrinking again. However, it does look as if gut bacteria could play a role in how we process elements of our diet and therefore could be part of the chain of internal events that leads to obesity. Just remember, though, that this internal chain of events is fuelled by what you put into your mouth.

The dolphin of consensus

The link between obesity and bacteria has been the subject of numerous studies in recent years and, as with much of what is discussed in this book, it can be difficult to form a clear picture from the confusing evidence and counter-evidence, theory and counter-theory, that is published seemingly constantly. Sometimes it feels like looking at one of those 3-D posters, when every so often a dolphin or a fairy castle comes sharply into focus, only to disappear and be replaced by cross-eyed chaos. The lure of an easy solution to obesity and the relevance of this to, sadly, so many people attract the media to such stories like a pack of ravening wolves around a weakened fawn. By the time they have digested the science and pooped it out there is frequently nothing left on which to hang any rational conclusion. However, the dolphin of consensus is starting to appear from the chaos of random colours.

A study that both strengthens and demonstrates the basics of the developing consensus was undertaken by scientists working in a trans-Atlantic collaboration between Cornell University and King's College London, led by Julia Goodrich. Their research used twins, specifically 171 pairs of identical twins and 245 pairs of non-identical twins, and more than a thousand samples of poo.[2]

Twin studies are a powerful technique for scientists trying to unravel the effects of genes, the environment and, in this case, the in-vironment. At their simplest, twin studies exploit the fact that identical twins are genetically identical while non-identical twins are not, and that both twins are likely to have similar nurturing environments. Scientists then use these genetic and environmental similarities and differences to analyse the variation observed and to work out the influence that genes, environment or a combination of both play in causing that variation.

There are complications to this paradigm. For example, in reality the effects of 'environment' can be exceptionally hard to identify and quantify. The holy grail of twin studies is a separated-at-birth identical-twin pair that can be reunited and studied in later life. Their genes are identical but their environment (their nurture, as opposed to their nature) has usually been enormously different. Understandably, such cases are rare, although not unknown. Also, although not necessarily a major problem for twin studies, identical twins are not in fact identical, a revelation that has nothing to do with bacteria but is interesting enough to warrant a deviation.

At the moment of conception, when a single egg is fertilised, it forms what is termed a zygote. This usually goes on to produce one embryo. Sometimes, however, it splits to form two zygotes, genetically identical, that go on to form two embryos. Hence, we get identical twins, also known as monozygotic ('one-zygote') twins. Non-identical twins come from two zygotes arising from two separately fertilised eggs and are thus known as dizygotic twins. However, from the point when the zygote splits, monozygotic twins are separate entities, subject to tiny differences in their environment within the womb and small, random differences in the way their bodies develop. These environmental differences result in different fingerprints, for example, but changes can also occur in the DNA within each twin.

As the single-celled zygote grows, cells divide and new copies of DNA must be made to populate these new cells. This mass copying of DNA results in small errors called somatic mutations (because they occur in the *soma* or body rather than in the sex cells, where they could be passed on to offspring). Mutations occurring early in development can, through cell division, end up in many of the cells of the final body and research suggests that a typical pair of identical twins have 359 of these early-development mutations separating them genetically and potentially leading to different genetic tendencies for diseases like cancer.[3]

But back to our thousand poo samples: the research team sequenced the genes of microbes present in these samples and compared the two types of twins. What they found was interesting and convenient because in one hit it sums up a great deal of what we know about gut bacteria and the link to obesity.

The gut community was more similar in identical than in non-identical twins and analysis showed that aspects of this community were influenced by the genetics of the person whose gut it was. This confirms other research that has demonstrated that when we talk about 'our' gut microbiota the sense of personal ownership is not misplaced. Although there is tremendous variation between people, and an individual's gut microbiota can and does change over time, there is a personal uniqueness to our internal community that is connected to our genes.

Internal stability

Stability is a tricky concept in ecology because it can be hard to define what we mean by stable. A traffic cone is the standard ecological analogy for stability and I am sure that the student obsession with them is driven by their desire to explore ecologically stable-state analogies. One meaning of stability is that a system resists change; in other words, we can mess about with it and it doesn't react, unless we give a really catastrophic shove, of course. Nothing is completely stable. A traffic cone standing on its base is the picture you should have in your mind at this point. You can knock the cone over but you need to put a fair amount of effort into it and under most circumstances the cone resists change and stays upright. So, is our gut an upright traffic cone? Well, we already know that taking antibiotics causes a change to our gut microbiota, so the system is not entirely resistant to change, but taking antibiotics amounts to a dramatic ecological disturbance akin to setting fire to a forest. Smaller disturbances like eating different foods seem to have almost no effect. So, to some extent, our gut microbiota can resist disturbance, but it can also be pushed over the edge in certain extreme circumstances.

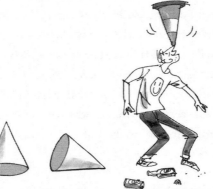

Stable cone   Neutral cone   Unstable cone

A system could also exhibit resilience, which is to say that it returns quickly to its previous state when disturbed. If we turn our traffic cone onto its side we get a similar state of stability. We can push the cone and it rolls around, but overall it remains in the same state: on its side. It may have shifted position, though. Testing people over time has shown that gut bacteria samples from the same individual are more similar to one another than samples from different individuals, but 'more similar' is not the same as 'identical'. Disturbances can indeed produce change (the traffic cone can shift), but there seems to be a stable, equilibrium state that our community is drawn towards.[4] The recovered-state gut microbiota, although functionally similar (it does the same job), will have lost or gained some species and they could be in different proportions than before the disturbance. Ecologically, we would say that the community is 'functionally resilient'.

Linking up bacteria and obesity

In the twin study, the bacterial family that had the most heritable component, in other words the bacteria most affected by the genetics of the person in whose bowel they were dwelling, was the Christensenellaceae. These bacteria occurred with other species forming what is called a co-occurrence network, or a reasonably stable 'core community' of species. Here's where things start getting really interesting, because this co-occurrence network was a more prominent component of the gut microbiota in people with lower BMIs. That's right: thin people had gut bacteria communities that were different to fat people's and components of those communities were heritable. This is, of course, a brilliant double roll-over jackpot of an excuse for obesity – 'it's my genes *and* my bacteria'!

The problem with this type of seductive story is that the evidence trail is correlative. The presence of certain bacteria correlates with being lean, but this doesn't necessarily mean that those bacteria are causing leanness or that their impoverishment could lead to obesity. There is a correlation between the number of spiders I have seen in my house over the last three autumns and the amount of coffee I am drinking, but there is clearly no causal relationship between my addiction and arachnids. In fact, more spiders were probably caused by moving house to a more rural location, a move that was provoked by an expanding family, which also explains the coffee drinking. In this case a third factor, family size, correlates with the other two observed phenomena and provides the causal factor for both. In science, to move from correlation to clear causal relationship typically requires what is called an interventional study or an experiment, when we do something to the system in question and study the effects of our interventions.

This is exactly what Goodrich and her colleagues carried out. They took an 'obese-associated microbiome' (which was, in reality, poo from a fat person) and added to that community a member of the Christensenellaceae family called *Christensenella minuta*. When ingested, this enrichment made the recipient's bacterial community more similar to that associated with lean people: in other words, it is possible to alter a person's microbiome to one associated with more or less desirable characteristics. The bacterially altered poo was also given to germfree mice (we met these in Chapters Six and Seven). What the researchers found was that those mice receiving *C. minuta* supplement had altered microbiotas and, crucially, gained less weight than those that didn't get the bacterial boost.[5]

If we consider these results without knowledge of the connection between the Christensenellaceae bacteria and obesity, they are mind-blowing. To cut to the chase, it indicates that eating the poo of someone thin could potentially help you to lose weight, or at least not to gain weight. A pretty horrible and ironically demeaning prospect, for sure, but mind-blowing nonetheless. When we are armed with knowledge of the reach and scope of our internal ecosystem, however, the notion that such an intervention could work seems at least credible. It is tempting to jump on such results and suggest that obesity can be 'cured' by ingesting *C. minuta*, but it is still early days and the support of evidence from germfree mice in laboratory conditions does not equate to a miracle cure for obesity. This study does, though, indicate that our genes can influence our microbiome and that the microbiome could play a role (as yet not fully unravelled) in our tendency to get fat.

Goodrich et al.'s study joins up some of the links in the evidence chain and certainly points towards a potential for 'bacterial therapy' in combating obesity. As might be expected, however, the picture is not as simple as the one I've painted. For a start, recent research suggests that diet may trump genes when it comes to gut microbiota. Consumption of a high-fat, high-sugar diet reproducibly altered the gut microbiota of study mice and a change in diet over only three and a half days was enough to change that microbiota community to a new stable state.[6] This was despite genetic differences between the individuals, but interestingly the change could be reversed with a change in diet. People still debate 'nature versus nurture', but this is largely a false dichotomy. So much of what we know points squarely to nature *and* nurture, and our gut bacteria are no different. Our genetics work with our environment, and what we shovel into our in-vironment, to affect our microbiota.

It's never simple . . .

Other studies indicate different roles for different bacteria. One such study examined the effect bacteria in the large intestine could have on the way we use fat. Fatty, or adipose, tissue is of two types in humans. White fat is the storage tissue that we collect under our skin and around our organs. Simply put, it's the stuff that makes us 'fat' and even in people who are not overweight there can be a fair bit of it about. Brown fat, on the other hand, is found in small deposits around the neck and upper chest and is involved not in energy storage but in generating heat, a function for which it is highly adapted. It is this heat production that leads to brown fat being more common in hibernating mammals and in newborn infants, who cannot generate heat by shivering. Crucially for our story, brown fat uses energy when it is stimulated, including energy locked up in white fat. So, from a horribly simplistic obesity-centric viewpoint, white fat is 'bad' and brown fat is 'good'.

The amounts of brown and white fat in different people vary and evidence suggests that lean people have relatively more brown fat than overweight and obese people. Comparing germfree mice (with no gut bacteria, remember) with normal mice, a team from Imperial College London and the Nestlé Research Centre in Switzerland found than brown fat in the germfree mice was more active and burned calories faster than in the normal mice. One reason why this could be happening is that an absence of bacteria means that carbohydrates are not being fermented to produce short-chain fatty acids (a process that we met back in Chapter Six) and this absence disrupts metabolic processes that eventually lead to calorie-burning in brown fat.[7] The therapeutic benefit of this knowledge is not immediately clear, but in the fight against global obesity it feels as if any knowledge is potential power. At a public demonstration of some early attempts at ballooning, when asked what the good of such a thing could be, Benjamin Franklin is alleged to have replied, 'What good is a newborn baby?' and I think this is a good thought to bear in mind. We never know where research might lead.

Benjamin Franklin – know-it-all

Benjamin Franklin, of course, was famous for bons mots. My favourite is 'Three can keep a secret if two of them are dead' but better known is 'An apple a day keeps the doctor away'. Franklin was a fan of apples, asking his wife to ship him barrels of them when he was overseas (Newtown, or Newton, Pippins were his favourite, apparently). A popular image of Franklin is of an older man who is, even by generous estimations, fat, but for much of his life Franklin was trim, even being described as 'muscular' by his biographer

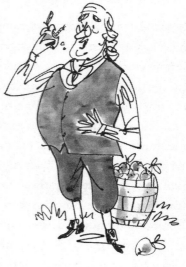

Walter Isaacson. Recent research into gut bacteria and obesity suggests that he may have been on to something with his 'apple a day' philosophy, but not perhaps in the way he might have thought.

Apple consumption has been linked with all sorts of medical benefits, including reducing the risk of heart disease, strokes and hypertension,[8] but a study published in 2014 made a surprising connection between apples, gut microbiota and obesity. This study examined the non-digestible components of apples, such as dietary fibre and polyphenols. Dietary fibre used to go by the name of roughage and consists of the indigestible components of plant-based food. Some dietary-fibre components are fermented in the gut by bacteria, while others resist any sort of breakdown and serve to bulk out our poo and ease its transit through the gut. Fibre is known to be prebiotic, which is to say it promotes the growth and activity of gut bacteria (more of which in Chapter Ten). Polyphenols are chemicals that contain large numbers (*poly*) of rings of carbon atoms bearing what chemists call a hydroxyl group (OH), a collection of atoms that is known as a phenol. They are important substances in plants and include the tannins found in bark, stems, fruit skin, leaf tissue and a cup of tea (where they contribute towards taste and colour).

The researchers induced obesity in mice by overfeeding them and then fed these fat mice a diet that included apples of different varieties. The poo of the fat mice was compared with that of the lean control mice in terms of bacterial composition. It was found that apple-fed fat mice had gut bacteria similar to those of lean mice, but different from those found in fat mice not fed apples. In other words, eating apples seemed to be altering the gut biota and promoting species associated with leanness.

The mechanism involves a process we have come across before: fermentation and the production of butyric acid. The fibre and polyphenol components of apples are being converted by bacteria into butyric acid that is promoting the growth of beneficial bacteria. The prebiotic effect of butyric acid has been noted by other researchers (and indeed suggested as a therapy for IBD[9]) and if you fancy doing a little self-medication then Granny Smiths were the variety with the best effect. Sadly, Franklin's Newtown Pippins were not part of the test.[10]

Playing God with your microbes

Manipulating an external environment to produce one that is more suited to our needs is commonplace. Indeed, it is the basis of agriculture and gardening. It makes perfect sense to take this environmental manipulation philosophy and apply it internally, altering our gut environment to allow beneficial bacterial species and communities to flourish at the expense of those causing problems. The approach underpins the probiotics and prebiotics discussed in Chapter Ten, but it is possible to play 'environmental architect' in more subtle ways than the pro- and prebiotic industry generally does.

Research in 2014 took just such a subtle approach. A safe strain of our old friend *E. coli* was taken and genetically modified so that it would produce substances going by the catchy chemical name of N-acetyl-phosphatidylethanolamines, abbreviated, thankfully, to NAPEs. NAPEs are lipids (fats) that are produced in our small intestine when we eat and converted rapidly to N-acylethanolamides, known as NAEs. These NAEs are involved in signalling within the body, telling it to reduce food intake, inhibit fat absorption and increase breakdown of fats and other processes that reduce obesity. The researchers gave one group of mice modified *E. coli* in their drinking water for eight weeks, while other groups received either inert bacteria (cells that were modified but then killed to control for the effects of giving bacteria to mice) or plain water. All mice were fed on a high-fat diet, with food they could access whenever they wanted, a regime known as *ad libitum* feeding. The group receiving the modified bacteria had significantly reduced food intake and body fat, as well as showing far less hepatic steatosis (or 'fatty liver'). Interestingly, the changes in gut microbiota brought about by the experiment remained for about six weeks after the modified bacteria had been removed from the drinking water, while the body weight and body fat benefits were still apparent 12 weeks after the modified *E. coli* were removed.[11]

The work is ongoing and researchers are, of course, pushing towards a therapeutic solution in humans rather than an experimental system in mice but, as we have seen, obesity is a complex problem and our gut bacteria are a complex community. That they should intersect in ways that suggest we are unlikely to find a single simple solution is to be expected, however nice the 'here's some bacteria, get them down your neck and look like Brad Pitt' solution would be. I think it is instructive to consider the thoughts of the senior researcher on the E. coli NAPE project, Sean Davies, of Vanderbilt University in Nashville, quoted in Medical News Today: 'Since it worked in mice eating a high-fat diet, it does suggest that it will be beneficial, even if people don't change their diet to something including more vegetables and less junk food. But we expect that it would likely provide the most benefit to those who do change their diet and try to get sufficient exercise.'[12] In other words, eating less and doing more are still the best interventions we have.

CHAPTER NINE

Why It's Good to Stay in Touch with 'Old Friends'

In which we consider the rise of allergies, cast aside the hygiene hypothesis, embrace old friends and learn the startling fact that gut bacteria might be affecting our mental health. Really ...

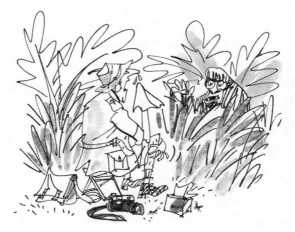

I take students on field trips and before we head off they are required to fill in a Health and Safety form. It's not an onerous task by any means, but it is a useful way to keep track of any medical conditions or dietary requirements that it might be better to know about in advance rather than to discover late at night in the South

African bush. It is by no means uncommon for these forms to list allergies of one form or another. These may be relatively benign, as with the student who was allergic to lobster (I'll be sure to mention it to the maître d'), but they may also include more troublesome conditions such as severe hay fever and these seem to be getting more common. Studies and surveys back up my observation. Allergies are indeed on the rise, with the charity Allergy UK suggesting that they will affect 30–35% of people at some point in their lives, and up to 50% of children being diagnosed with an allergic condition.

Asthma also makes a regular appearance on these forms. A long-term and distressing inflammatory disease, asthma affects the airways and for many sufferers attacks are triggered by an allergic reaction to something 'out there' in the environment, such as pollen, animal fur, cigarette smoke or dust mites, or by exercise. Not all sufferers have allergic triggers, but non-allergic, or intrinsic, asthma, is less common than the allergic, or extrinsic, kind. The allergen (the agent causing the allergic response) initiates a complex reaction in the body that results in an over-the-top inflammatory response by the immune system. The resulting inflamed and swollen airways and lungs cause coughing, wheezing, shortness of breath, chest tightness and breathing troubles. These deeply unpleasant symptoms are largely reversible with medication, such as salbutamol, administered through an inhaler.

That I should be seeing more asthma on Health and Safety forms is not surprising. In the UK, where most of my students come from, more than five million people (one in twelve adults and one in eleven children) currently receive treatment for this disease. When I was a child there was perhaps one pupil per class carrying an exotic-looking blue inhaler (which it turns out isn't 'recreational', so don't bother), but over the last decade or so the number of asthma sufferers in Western Europe has doubled and similar rises are reported in the US and Australia.[1] The developing world has also seen an increase in asthma and the rise cannot be associated with increased recognition or treatment of the disease: asthma is not difficult to recognise and salbutamol has been a first-line treatment since the late 1960s. The rises we are seeing in allergies and asthma are real; the obvious question to ask is why?

The hygiene hypothesis

We have already seen that a tight and important connection exists between our bacterial microbiota and our immune system. The adaptive 'teachable' component of our immune system develops as a consequence of exposure to potential bacterial friends and foes. An allergic response can be thought of as the result of poor learning; the immune system has trouble distinguishing between friend and foe and overreacts, taking us back to the analogy we saw in Chapter Seven, of some kind of overzealous nightclub bouncer beating seven bells out of everyone who tries to get through the door. If we extend this line of thinking a little, we end up with a hypothesis for the rise in allergies that has attracted considerable attention in the media and has tended to inform the public's understanding of the subject: the 'hygiene hypothesis'. As we will see, things are not all they seem with this seductively simple, and extremely persistent, explanation.

Declining infections in childhood and increases in allergic diseases were first linked in the 1970s. The idea that growing up in a farming environment, with its presumed greater opportunity for microbial exposure, could protect against hay fever and allergies had also gained ground. However, the 'hygiene hypothesis' as we know it really took off after a study by David Strachan in 1989. He was interested primarily in the rise in the prevalence of hay fever and in a *British Medical Journal* paper entitled 'Hay fever, hygiene and household size' he put forward an elegant suggestion to account for this rise, and the rises observed in asthma and childhood eczema. He wrote: 'Over the past century declining family size, improvements in household amenities, and higher standards of personal cleanliness have reduced the opportunity for cross infection in young families. This may have resulted in more widespread clinical expression of atopic disease [*those causing hypersensitive allergic reactions – commonly hay fever, eczema and asthma*], emerging earlier in wealthier people, as seems to have occurred for hay fever.' In other words, unhygienic contact with siblings, allowing for the spread of infection, is a 'good' thing in terms of avoiding allergies, despite the resulting infections one might acquire.[2]

This hypothesis subsequently gained traction in the popular press, possibly because it seems so refreshingly straightforward and logical. It also plays directly into the hands of those who enjoy a little intergenerational one-upmanship. It runs like this.

In the 'good old days' allergies and asthma were uncommon. In those days children played outside more and came into contact far more with animals, plants and soil. We were also less concerned with hygiene in the home (a bit damning to our forebears and difficult to test without a time machine) and we lacked the arsenal of antibacterial products that we so assiduously deploy these days. Consequently, in these mythical good old days, not only were Mars Bars the size of house bricks, but we also had plenty of exposure to microorganisms in our 'filthy' homes and by God our immune systems prospered. Those immune systems learnt until they could learn no more. They were the PhDs of immune systems and sure, we may have died from TB and dysentery, but at least we could eat nuts. These days, of course, everyone is weak, sniffling and wheezing through the streets with their allergies and asthma. The modern immune system is cut off from its bacterial lecturers because we are all so damn hygienic and kids never get to eat dirt like they did back then.

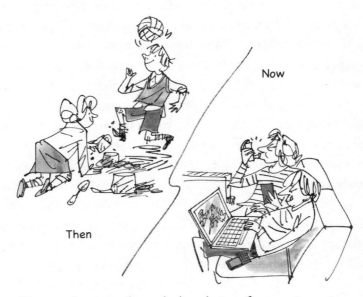

It's a seductive tale and the chain of reasoning seems to have merit. Certainly, knowing what we do about immunity and bacteria, it does not seem illogical to suggest that a lack of exposure to bacteria early in life, particularly low-level 'background' or 'subclinical' exposure, could cause problems with our immune system's development. That the hypothesis has biological plausibility is one of its great strengths. However, it's a big step from a seductive idea and some interesting correlations to a scientific consensus on a proven causal relationship.

Are we really that clean?

It's interesting that our concerns about bacteria in our homes are so horribly contradictory. On the one hand we can't do enough, or spend enough, to eradicate them and on the other hand we worry that we've done too good a job. We can't have it both ways and to get things in perspective it is worth thinking back to Chapters Two and Three and the great practical difficulties of killing bacteria in all those complex three-dimensional environments like the bathroom and kitchen. Is it really likely that we are keeping our homes *so* clean, *so* devoid of bacterial life, that the resulting domestic dead zone is affecting our children's health? After all, we can't even wash our hands properly most of the time (Chapter Four). Your gut feeling has to be 'no', and in fact clean homes were never supposed to be a part of the explanation.

Strachan's paper focused on the inverse relationship between family size and allergic disorders, primarily hay fever. An inverse relationship describes situations where one value increases (in this case hay fever) while the other (family size) decreases. Strachan linked this relationship to the higher levels of cross-infection that are possible in larger families, noting that a reduction in family size (typically seen in developed nations) could result in reduced cross-infection and increased allergies. He also noted that 'improvements in household amenities, and higher standards of personal cleanliness' could reduce the opportunity for cross-infection and with these ten words the 'hygiene hypothesis' as we now know it formed.

However, Strachan did not specifically state that our homes are now so clean that our children's immune systems are not exposed to any bacteria and that's why they have increased allergies. He suggested instead that smaller families were a key factor and then speculated that better household amenities and improved personal hygiene *might* be important. Nowhere in this original paper was 'home hygiene' explicitly mentioned, although clearly one could make that inference. And many did.

The hygiene hypothesis became an umbrella term within science for a range of ideas concerning the links between microbial exposure and the prevalence of allergic diseases like asthma, eczema and hay fever. The problem is that in the popular media those complex factors have become distilled into a single, easy-to-grasp concept: our homes are too clean. So, what evidence is there to support all this?

Have we really become too clean for our own good?

A considerable amount of research has examined the different issues that come under the 'hygiene hypothesis' umbrella and the most consistent findings are: that there is a decreasing risk of atopic diseases (particularly hay fever) for people from families with three or more siblings; and that there is a decreasing risk for younger siblings, particularly if older siblings are brothers.[3] The relationship between family size and allergic diseases that was suggested by the original data has been supported by some studies, but the findings are not entirely consistent when individual diseases are examined.[4]

However, findings about family size or family structure do not lend any support *at all* to the notion that our homes are too clean, and neither could they. To do that requires us to examine and measure home and personal hygiene and to quantify the health of the people in those homes. Scientifically, the ideal solution would be to manipulate hygiene in homes, but such a study is likely to fall foul of the ethics committee. If we ask people to be less hygienic then we know, for a fact, that they are likely to suffer health costs from increased potential infections and if we ask them to be more hygienic then we have some reason to suppose they could end up with more allergies (since this is the basis of the hypothesis we are testing). Another approach, albeit correlative, would be to look at the use of cleaning products and practices and at the prevalence of allergies across space (comparing different countries, perhaps) and time.

A number of studies have examined the potential causal link between our supposedly clean modern homes and the rise of allergies. If you are one of those people who have been moaning about how our clean homes are giving us allergies, then I am afraid it's time to brace yourself for a nasty shock…

The hygiene hypothesis doesn't really work

Overall, studies examining the possible link between home hygiene and allergic diseases have pretty much drawn a blank. The link simply doesn't exist. Yes, we are using more cleaning products now than before, but consumption overall or for specific types of products in different European countries has no correlation with the rise in allergic diseases when other factors are controlled for. Bacteria, as we have seen, are remarkably good at recolonising surfaces and multiplying rapidly; in reality our cleaning habits, even if they do involve the latest fancy cleaning product, do little to stop that. Some practices can even increase the distribution of bacteria around the home. Maybe a knife that has cut raw chicken is wiped with a cloth that is later used to wipe down the worktop? I think I'm reasonably careful with domestic hygiene and yet

I catch myself making small but potentially significant lapses in procedure all the time. I know that I would rather jump into a time machine and eat food off my grandmother's clean and bleached kitchen work surfaces than graze from my own, cursorily wiped with a contaminated cloth and some aggressively branded 'wonder cleaner'.

In a major review of the hygiene hypothesis published in 2006, the conclusion was extremely clear: 'Evidence of a link between atopy [*diseases like hay fever, eczema and asthma*] and domestic cleaning and hygiene is weak at best'.[5] In fact, the authors go a little further in their summary, stating that the 'increase in allergic disorders does not correlate with the decrease in infection with pathogenic organisms [*those causing disease*], *nor can it be explained by changes in domestic hygiene* [my emphasis]'. A second major review of the hypothesis was published in 2012.[6] Freely available online, it's a technical but approachable review that I thoroughly recommend you read if you want to understand more about the hygiene hypothesis and its implications. The authors of this review go one step further, stating that 'the idea that "poor hygiene in itself would be protective" [*in other words, that a dirty house protects your children from allergies*] is now generally refuted' and adding, one senses wearily, 'although it is still discussed in the popular media'.

The simple 'hygienic home' hypothesis was, and is, so seductive that it has proved to have remarkable longevity in the press and the public's perceptions, long past the point where this simple formulation has any scientific validity. It is so seductive, in fact, that many people ignore clear problems in the logic. We have seen already that our homes abound with microorganisms no matter how much cleaning we do. Also, the notion that the modern home is any cleaner now than it was 30 or 40 years ago is hard to justify. Given our more hectic lifestyle and the move away from a domestic model where one partner (virtually always the woman) remained at home to 'keep house', I would suggest that a logical position to maintain would be that our homes are far *less* hygienic than they were.[7] I know mine is.

Integral to the hygiene hypothesis, or at least to many people's interpretation of it, is the idea that children don't play outdoors as much and so are not exposed to microbes out there either. Again, a seductive idea (albeit one that needs evidential support), but surely a consequence of children not being outdoors is that they spend more time indoors, and I can pretty much guarantee they aren't cleaning. Wouldn't this again make for *less* hygienic homes?

The hygiene hypothesis is dead; long live the microbial deprivation hypothesis?

The term 'hygiene hypothesis', so firmly centred on home cleanliness, is misleading and unhelpful. These days, scientific papers that mention it usually do so either to suggest that it is no longer used (like the teacher shouting at pupils to be quiet in the library, a slightly contradictory position in which to find yourself) or as a part of some introductory, historical scene-setting. However, the death of the simplistic 'clean house' model does not spell the end for the entangled concepts sheltering beneath the hygiene hypothesis umbrella. In fact, the basic concept of a link between microbial exposure and allergic disease is accepted and has become the consensus.

Returning to Strachan's original formulation, the link between allergy and infection is based on the assumption that family size is a realistic proxy measure of infection. Proxy measures are measures of things we can quantify that we take as being representative of something that we can't. To make a wider inference, family size could also be a proxy measure for exposure to microbes in general. Scientifically, the hygiene hypothesis rapidly evolved from these early beginnings into the far broader notion that our modern lifestyles cause a decline in our exposure to microbes and a related increase in allergic disease through an impoverishment of learning opportunities for our immune systems. This enhanced 'Hygiene Hypothesis 2.0' embraced exposure to non-pathogenic bacteria, including species found in the wider environment, components of bacteria such as the toxins they can produce, and lifestyle issues that reduce microbial exposure, including the increase in urban living, reduction of contact with the 'environment' and with animals, and the decline of familial bed sharing. Proposals for a less misleading term that encompasses this enhanced understanding have included the 'microbial hypothesis' and the 'microbial deprivation hypothesis'.[8] Another related but subtly different explanation, the 'old friend hypothesis' has also gained considerable ground over the last few years.

These scientific advances, which I will discuss in a moment, have not attracted much attention within the media. Instead, the term 'hygiene hypothesis' is still widely used and has become shorthand for the alarmist and flagellatory message that 'we are doing too much home cleaning, our kids don't eat enough dirt and we're making them ill!'. This shorthand is outdated, simplistic, scientifically unsupported and potentially dangerous. It is dangerous because the implicit message of the hygiene hypothesis as commonly understood is that we would do better to relax our hygiene standards and in reality nothing could be further from the truth. As it is, poor hygiene standards, in kitchens especially, cause an immense amount of suffering and death. To lower those inadequate standards still further because it might mean little Johnny doesn't get asthma is scientifically unsupported madness. So, the next time you hear someone talking about how our clean homes are making kids ill and we should clean a lot less, please put them right.

Microbial exposure can be 'good'

Although the simplistic 'we clean too much' version of the hygiene hypothesis does not hold water, the fundamental fact that microbial exposure can be 'good' for us is valid. But how much and what sort of exposure is good, and why are we somehow having less of this beneficial exposure than we were in the past? We know now that home hygiene is a red herring, but we are left with the inescapable fact that microbial exposure comes from the environment and also via our in-environment. This logically leads to the conclusion that exposure to environmental microbes via our everyday lives and through our diet must somehow be important in developing, or not developing, our immune systems. We also know that exposure to some microbes is most definitely bad, while other microbes are common in and on our bodies and in many cases are beneficial, especially if they are a component of a balanced microbial community.

Furthermore, it is an inescapable fact that our lifestyles are very different now from what they were even 50 years ago. The changes that have happened have done so in the blink of an eye if we think in evolutionary time. Urbanisation and industrialisation fundamentally and dramatically alter the way we live and such alterations have clear benefits: we have more leisure time; we are less beholden to the vagaries of nature; and we have access to healthcare. There are also costs. For example, as early as the nineteenth century,

European physicians noted that farmers rarely suffered allergies, whereas hay fever was the mark of being a wealthy, well-educated member of the city élite. Urbanisation has continued apace and we are now an urban species, focused on indoor activities and fuelling them with a more processed diet. No amount of weekending in yurts and foraging in hedgerows is going to change that.

The Karelian peoples of Northern Europe provide an example of the sort of correlative evidence that helps to build the case for a connection between lifestyle (environment in a broader sense) and immunity-related diseases, not only hay fever and asthma but also IBD (Chapter Seven) and autoimmune diseases such as multiple sclerosis and, in this case, type 1 diabetes. Autoimmune diseases are characterised by an abnormal response of the immune system to substances and tissues normally found in the body (which gives us the *auto* or 'self' component of the name). We first met these diseases back in Chapter Three (Guillain-Barré Syndrome) and again in Chapter Seven, where we also met the regulatory T-cells (Treg) that usually prevent the immune system from reacting to the body's own cells and attacking them.

Ethnic Karelian people living in Russia have very low levels of type 1 diabetes and yet right over the border in Finland, at the same latitude, there is a six-fold increase in its incidence. This increase occurs against a near identical genetic background: in other words the Karelians in Russia and those in Finland are not 'different' ethnic groups lazily categorised as the same; they are genetically the same population, albeit one that has split recently as a consequence of politics into two subpopulations that rarely mix. There simply hasn't been enough time to generate significant genetic differences between these recently divergent subpopulations and yet there is a *six-fold* increase in the incidence of type 1 diabetes! If it's not caused by genetics, such a difference can only be a consequence of a different environment. In Russia the Karelians live in underdeveloped settlements in relative poverty, whereas in Finland (mostly in a region called North Karelia) the population is modernised and urbanised. A major difference between the two groups is that in Finland the exposure to microbes is far less than in the 'closer-to-nature' part of Russia in which the Russian Karelians live.[9]

The new challenger – the old friends hypothesis

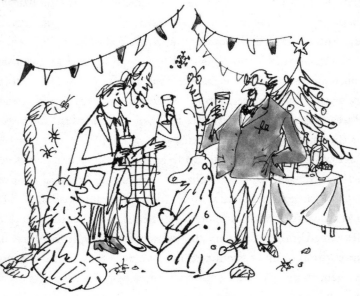

Reconciling what we know of the immune system and microbial exposure with lifestyle changes is clearly a challenge, but emerging from the hygiene hypothesis debate comes a new candidate: the 'old friends' or OF hypothesis. This was proposed by Graham Rook and colleagues in a paper published in 2004 entitled 'Mycobacteria and other environmental organisms as immunomodulators for immunoregulatory disorders'.[10] In this paper, the authors develop an argument that draws together the microbe-immunity-lifestyle connections in a far more satisfying way than the hygiene hypothesis. It's also got a catchier name, so it's something of a mystery that it remains relatively low profile. The argument goes as follows.

In the wealthy developed world there has been a steady and simultaneous rise in allergies (including hay fever), inflammatory bowel diseases including Crohn's disease and ulcerative colitis, and autoimmune diseases like multiple sclerosis and type 1 diabetes. There is evidence that these increases are at least partly attributable to malfunction of regulatory T-cells, a concept that we met in Chapter Seven in the context of IBD. Rook and colleagues surveyed the existing work and concluded that the increasing failure of regulatory T-cells is a consequence of reduced exposure to microorganisms that have had a continuous presence in the environment of mammals throughout their evolutionary history. They called these microbes our 'old friends', hence the OF hypothesis.

Immune systems, in us and in other mammals, did not evolve over the last few hundred years. The human immune system developed in our most distant human ancestors, itself building upon the immune system that had evolved in more distant, non-human ancestors. Our ancestral, evolutionary environment was the real, dirty, biodiverse world 'out there' and our relationship with it would have been intimate. Contact with mud and soil would have been inevitable, as would contact with the microorganisms dwelling within them, and within the faeces of animals and our fellow humans. These microorganisms include parasitic worms (flat worms and nematodes) and viruses as well as bacteria. As we gathered leaves and berries and ate them unwashed (shudder!), and hunted animals that we processed with our bare hands (what savages!), our contact with microorganisms was frequent, biodiverse and absolutely guaranteed.

Against this background of constant potential invaders our ancestral immune system had a big problem. It needed to respond to threats, but it would be inefficient and undesirable to react to absolutely everything. Firstly, such an 'all-in' response comes with a considerable cost to the bearer of that immune system, as we see in those suffering from allergies and inflammatory diseases. Secondly, components of our symbiotic microbiota are important to us and were important to our evolutionary forebears, but the overzealous bouncer ends up guarding an empty nightclub. Our immune system needs to be tolerant of organisms that are so common they can't be avoided and of those that are beneficial to us. We have evolved with these organisms, these 'old friends', and now we have evolved dependence on them to regulate aspects of our immune system. We need them to teach our immune system to walk the delicate tightrope between too much and too little; without their help the immune systems overbalances and falls. It isn't exposure in general, but specific exposure to these 'old friend' microorganisms that is the key.[11]

Old friends could wield much influence ...

IBD, allergies, asthma, eczema, hay fever, type 1 diabetes, multiple sclerosis: these are all inflammation-associated disorders and the OF hypothesis goes a long way towards explaining why we have seen increases in their prevalence and incidence. It may also have broader implications. Long-term inflammation can trigger cancer, and some types of cancers (such as Hodgkin's lymphoma, childhood lymphatic leukaemia, and colorectal and prostate cancer) show patterns of increase related to urbanisation that are similar to those seen in conditions like asthma. If the triggering inflammation occurs as a consequence of an immune system that has not been primed appropriately by old friends, then the connection to our health becomes even more significant.[12]

As our knowledge advances, and as we develop a more integrated and interconnected understanding of the relationship between us and microorganisms such as bacteria, we may uncover unexpected links. We saw in Chapter Seven that gut bacteria may be linked to anxiety in mice and there may be a relationship with depression in humans via the 'old friends' network'. Depression is, in a large group of patients, associated with an increase in cytokines. These small proteins are important in the complex system of communication that happens throughout our bodies at a cellular level. Signalling is a fascinating area of biology that happens within and between cells as well as the more familiar signalling that occurs between individuals. A honeybee worker that stings you releases a chemical signal, and this alarm pheromone changes the behaviour of other workers, causing them to come and sting you too. Cytokines are similar to pheromones, but act between cells, being released by some and changing the behaviour of others. Some cytokines are involved with immune responses and inflammation and if they are used clinically they can trigger depression in patients. There is also evidence that anti-inflammatory treatments can be effective against depression, which leads to some interesting speculation on the potential role of 'old friends' in our mental health, albeit speculation that must be exceptionally cautious and continually qualified with the important caveat that 'this research is at a very early stage'.[13]

The gut–mind connection

Research is revealing other intriguing connections between our gut bacteria and our mental state. For example, when researchers colonised the intestines of a timid strain of germfree mice with bacteria taken from the intestines of a bolder, more daring mouse strain, the recipient animals became more daring, exploring their environment. The opposite happened when the microbiota donation was reversed, with bold mice receiving timid mice's microbiota. The message here, though not one that is yet fully understood, is that microbial interactions with the brain could induce and maintain anxiety and mood disorders, as has already been suggested in IBS (see Chapter Seven).

We are also beginning to explore the potential role of gut microbiota in autism. Never was the caveat 'this research is at a very early stage' more appropriate, and it requires a few connections to be made along the way, but it is certainly encouraging. Epidemiological data has revealed that women who experience a high and prolonged fever during pregnancy are up to seven times more likely to have a child with autism. Researchers stimulated a fever state in pregnant germfree mice and the resulting offspring displayed limited social interactions, a tendency towards repetitive behaviour and reduced communication, which are three core symptoms of human autism. They also had 'leaky intestines', which is especially interesting since between 40 and 90% of children with autism also have gastrointestinal symptoms. When the researchers examined the gut microbiota of mice with and without these autism-like induced symptoms they found differences. The mice displaying autism symptoms had abnormal gut bacterial communities, with two classes of bacteria (the Clostridia and the Bacteroidia) being far more abundant than normal. When mice were dosed with *Bacteroides fragilis*, a bacterium known for its anti-inflammatory properties, the gut microbiota was pushed towards a more normal community, the intestinal leaks were fixed and the mice were less likely to be repetitive and uncommunicative. In other words, in mice, autism-like symptoms were reversed using a probiotic approach (of which we shall hear more in Chapter Ten). We are a long way from a probiotic solution to human autism, and such a solution could turn out to be impossible, but nonetheless scientists are now becoming convinced that our internal ecosystem has a potentially profound effect on our state of mind.[14]

We are used to the idea that *our* genes, encoded in the DNA in *our* cells, are what are important to *us*, but the OF hypothesis presents us with a startling reality. To function correctly our immune systems rely on genes present in other organisms, the genes that direct their development and function and give them the chemical properties that enable our immune systems to recognise them. Such organisms include not just bacteria but a wide range of micro-biodiversity such as nematode worms. Our modern lives reduce the opportunities for a regular get-together with these old friends, but it is wise not to force friendships. Encouraging your children to eat soil (as I have heard scientifically literate mothers suggesting more than once) or not to wash their hands after playing with the dog is not the way to go. Encouraging your child to play naturally outside and to engage with the natural world from an early age, on the other hand, could have an advantage, and not just for their immune system.

CHAPTER TEN

Are You Really Going To Eat That?

In which we consider the potentially confusing world of pre- and probiotics, the complexity of food labelling and the effectiveness of faecal microbiota transplants. Or poo-eating. Seriously, it works for some things. Honestly . . .

There's no doubt that I'd rather spend a sunny hour in one than the other but, despite that, gardens and guts are more similar than you might think. If we exclude the odd bit of storm damage and the pile of items we can't cram into the wheelie bin (I'm talking gardens here, by the way, although emergency-room reports about misplaced objects might suggest otherwise), then most of the problems with the average garden, and indeed gut, are biological.

Even if you don't have a plant-based garden, preferring things to be more clinical and life-free, then the first problem will be familiar: 'life' in the wrong place. Weeds that add a cheeky bit of colour to a family lawn spoil the lines of your lovingly laid deck and prod suggestively through the artificial grass. A bramble, once such a welcome natural screen, becomes a bloodthirsty tangle of thorny whips scourging everyone that passes. Weedkiller provides a rapid and effective solution but, if carelessly applied, then, like antibiotics thrown into the gut community, it can cause collateral damage.

Pest is really just a word for 'life in the wrong place' and an organism is only considered to be a pest when it causes a problem, perhaps because of lost income from crops or decreased attractiveness of the garden. Items on the long list of organisms we consider pests, from fungi to foxes via aphids and wasps, like bacteria in soil or animal faeces, are not pests most of the time. It's only when too many of them end up on our roses, or in our gut, that the problems start.

Killing pests is often quite easy. Insects, for example, are common pests of agricultural crops and there are a number of very effective chemicals that will wipe out most of them. However, there are all sorts of issues that can result from using such chemicals. Wholesale use of insecticides might end up killing off your pest's natural enemies. This means that when the insecticide has disappeared the pest can re-establish with no natural enemies at all, something known as target pest resurgence. When you are dealing with communities of interacting organisms, at whatever physical scale, interfering with one 'harmful' component can have unpredictable and undesirable consequences on harmless or even useful components. There might also be predictable effects. Just as bacteria evolve resistance to antibiotics, so some pests can evolve resistance to pesticides, especially if they are used incorrectly or indiscriminately.

The history of pest management is interesting to compare with the emerging understanding of our microbiota and its management. After the Second World War the chemical industry hit something of a purple patch when it came to developing and marketing chemicals for killing pests, especially insects and plants. The 1950s were the golden age of chemical pest control in agriculture and there is no denying that the benefits in terms of increased crop yields were immense. The costs, though, also became apparent. Collateral environmental damage, ramified and magnified through complex food webs, led to a dramatic decrease in birds vulnerable to the eggshell-thinning effects of the insecticide DDT, for example. Recently, we have started to unravel the unwanted effects of neonicotinoid insecticides on bees, but that is really just the latest in a succession of the 'product-problem-prohibition' cycle that has characterised chemical pest control. The comparison with our microbiota is obvious: the 'bacteria = bad' model has led to an overuse of, and an overreliance on, antibiotics, with two major effects. Firstly, antibiotics cluster-bomb our gut microbiota and, secondly, the harmful bacteria we seek to destroy have, in many cases, evolved resistance.

Modern pest control has moved away from the 'spray and pray' philosophy towards what has become known as integrated pest management or IPM. This is an ecologically intelligent and effective system that does not shun chemicals where appropriate, but seeks to combine them with biological and physical means of controlling pests in ways that are environmentally sustainable. A typical IPM approach might be to improve the habitat around crops to encourage the natural enemies of target pests to thrive. Such improvement might include installing nest boxes in the trees around crop fields. These boxes encourage the presence of hungry broods of chicks in need of constant filling with just the sort of caterpillars that are ravaging the crop below.

Recently we have seen an IPM type of philosophy emerge in the way we think about our microbiota, especially our gut bacteria. Rather than simplistically 'seeking to destroy' we are now investigating, and indeed regularly using, means to nurture or to re-establish healthy gut microbial communities. In this way, we act like sensitive, ecologically informed managers of our in-vironment. This approach is encapsulated in two sometimes controversial concepts that differ by only one letter, but whose modes of action differ radically: prebiotics and probiotics.

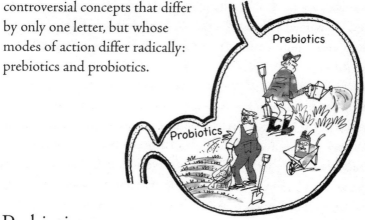

Prebiotics – feeding your internal lawn

Prebiotics encourage the growth and activity of our microbiota. In general, prebiotics are concerned with nurturing bacteria in the gut, and this is certainly where the bulk of the research and commercial interest is focused. In principle, though, there is no reason why other components of our microbiota cannot be encouraged for the improvement of our health. There are prebiotic moisturisers and hand creams available, for example, although reading through information about some of these products suggests to me that a little bandwagon-jumping has been going on. One product, by REN Skincare, is advertised as a prebiotic hand cream yet contains the baffling publicity statement that it contains 'prebiotics to protect and stimulate the skin *against* bacteria [my emphasis]'. Whatever that might mean, and frankly I don't know, the product certainly doesn't seem to be prebiotic in any scientific sense of the word.

Another 'prebiotic' product that caught my eye also caught the ever-vigilant eye of the US Food and Drug Administration (the FDA). The interestingly branded 'Luvena Vaginal Moisturizer', manufactured by Laclede Incorporated, is sold over the counter with claims that it soothes, refreshes and lubricates (presumably the vagina, although this isn't actually made clear on the box). These claims do seem to be backed up with good customer feedback on third-party sites, but the efficacy or otherwise of the product is not the reason the FDA issued an injunction against Laclede in January 2015. The problem was the company's use of the words 'prebiotic' and 'actibiotic', the latter being a word that appears to be found solely in association with commercial products, tests on commercial products, patents and FDA injunctions. It is used interchangeably with prebiotic but with the added advantage (at least if you are trying to pitch your product as vaguely 'medical') of being easily confused with antibiotic. One firm, Vitamin Research Products, actually claims to own ActiBiotic as a trademark on some of its products. Far be it from me to dispense advice on legal matters, but VRP's lawyers really need to get busy and start billing some hours, because the term is thrown around with scant regard for any ownership by a diverse array of those operating on the snake-oil side of the cosmetics and supplements market.

The term 'prebiotic', at least according to the FDA and, if we are honest, to common sense, makes medical implications about a product. The FDA declared that Laclede Incorporated was 'in violation of the Federal Food, Drug, and Cosmetic Act for introducing unapproved and improperly labelled (misbranded) drugs for sale across the country'. You can sell a vaginal moisturiser if you want, but if you make claims about enzymes nurturing bacteria, and if you use words like prebiotic, then the FDA take the stance that you are selling a drug. The injunction prevents Laclede from marketing 'any products that contain the term "prebiotic" or "actibiotic" on its labels or packages without obtaining the FDA's approval'.[1]

Dietary prebiotics are more straightforward in some respects. Non-digestible fibre, a type of carbohydrate that we met when discussing apples and obesity in Chapter Eight, is what we generally mean when we talk about dietary prebiotics, and the concept that these substances can be prebiotic was introduced in 1995.[2]

Carbohydrates consist of chains of sugars linked together and, in the case of prebiotics, there are three types. Short-chain prebiotics are smaller molecules that are mostly fermented in the right-side, or ascending, colon, whereas long-chain molecules are mostly fermented in the left-side, or descending, colon; full-spectrum prebiotics are a mixture of both types. The fermentation of prebiotics, as we have already seen, produces short-chain fatty acids and other substances that are beneficial to the bacteria dwelling within the gut and may, in some cases, be absorbed to give benefits in the wider body. Of course, we want not just to help bacteria generally, but to ensure that beneficial bacteria get the most help. Of these beneficial bacteria, prebiotics most often assist two groups that are common in the gut ecosystem, the lactobacillae and, more significantly in most cases, the bifidobacteria.

Prebiotic fibre

Prebiotic fibre can be found widely in fruit, vegetables, pulses and grains. Chicory root is the current prebiotic chart topper, but you don't need to go down the 'obscure vegetables' aisle to make sure you have some in your diet. Here are some other rich sources[3]:

Blueberry, pear, watermelon

Spring onion, leek, white onion

Jerusalem artichoke, garlic

Also, asparagus, sugar beet, wheat, honey, banana, barley, tomato, rye, lentils, peas, beans, chickpeas and mustard.[4]

Cooked onions, bananas, apples, beans, unrefined grains, leeks, artichokes, asparagus, garlic, cabbage and root vegetables are all great sources of prebiotics. Oh, hang on a minute; I've just described a balanced diet ...

Of course, a big problem is that many of us don't have an especially balanced diet and may have some health problems connected to our microbiota. We possibly also lack sufficient contact with the 'old friends' we met in Chapter Nine. Obvious health problems include the inflammatory bowel diseases (discussed in Chapter Seven), obesity (Chapter Eight) and allergic diseases (Chapter Nine), but might also take in lower-level symptoms indicative of poor gut health and, potentially, of a poorly balanced bacterial community. I guess we can take our pick here from bloating, constipation, cramps and diarrhoea.

With new discoveries about the role of our gut and other bacterial communities being made all the time, we are entering a period where many health issues might soon have a firm scientific connection to our microbiota confirmed and explored for therapeutic options. Given our tendency to seek out the easiest solution to any problem, prebiotic supplements or adding prebiotics directly to food feel like obvious steps forward and considerably less trouble than prescribing a balanced diet rich in fruit and vegetables, despite the additional health benefits such a lifestyle change would entail. But do prebiotics really bring any benefit?

There is very good evidence supporting the effectiveness of prebiotics.[5] Added to specific foodstuffs or taken orally, they have been shown to have positive health benefits in a number of 'human feeding studies'. Two groups of prebiotic substances in particular, the galactans and the fructans, have been shown to be effective in increasing the levels of bifidobacteria. Research has tended to focus on these prebiotics, and on bifidobacteria, but as our understanding of the gut microbiota increases we will undoubtedly see more potential prebiotic targets (and prebiotic substances) being investigated. We will also see the picture becoming more complex than just 'helping good bacteria'. In a fast-moving and exciting field there is evidence that prebiotics could help in combating obesity[6] and that the fermentation of prebiotics might help to steer the immune system towards an anti-inflammatory state because the products produced by fermentation affect the permeability of the intestine.[7]

The idea of supplementing our food with added prebiotics is appealing. Many of us do not eat a diet naturally rich in such substances and if we know that there is a benefit, and that they can be added easily and without affecting the taste, then shouldn't we do just that? Before we do, it is important to remember that the benefits of prebiotics are supported by human feeding studies taking place under controlled laboratory conditions as part of a carefully monitored diet. They might support the use of a given prebiotic, but that does not mean that we should start adding galacto-oligosaccharides or anything else to our food because 'it's good for us'. Adding prebiotics to food, indeed adding anything to food, is controversial and rightly so. It needs to be proved that adding prebiotics would be good for us in the real world, when mixed in with the many different chemicals in our food and ingested as part of a realistic diet. The evidence is growing, and very encouraging, but it is still early days.

Probiotics – replanting your internal lawn

Prebiotics are all about managing your in-vironment to make it a place in which beneficial gut bacteria can thrive, essentially by providing them with something to 'eat'. A better definition is that a prebiotic is a selectively fermented ingredient that results in changes to the composition and/or activity of the gut microbiota and a subsequent benefit to health. To return to our garden analogy, it's like chucking manure on your roses. A *probiotic* approach, on the other hand, doesn't aim to encourage existing beneficial bacteria, but instead seeks to introduce those bacteria directly. Rather than chucking manure on the roses, probiotic strategies plant more roses. They are also a little bit like chucking manure down your own throat, sometimes less analogically and more literally than you might realise.

It is not surprising that, even in the very early days of the probiotic approach, yogurt was the food of choice. Milk is converted into yogurt through the fermentation action of specific types of bacteria that convert lactose (the 'milk sugar' that some people have problems digesting) into lactic acid. We also produce lactic acid by a form of fermentation called anaerobic respiration, which is especially important during intense exertion because it can supply our muscles with the energy they need more rapidly than aerobic respiration. The lactic acid we produce when we have to rely on anaerobic respiration, like when we sprint, accumulates in our muscles and causes soreness that requires plenty of deep breathing and a gin and tonic to cure. The lactic acid that yogurt-producing bacteria create, rather than causing soreness, gives yogurt an acidic tang and causes proteins in the milk to change their shape and thicken up the mixture. Yogurt is a bacterial product.

The father of probiotics

Probiotics aren't new. The concept of a radical reintroduction campaign to restore the community balance of gut microbiota was actually first proposed by, or more accurately first attributed to, the Russian Nobel Prize-winning biologist Ilya Ilyich Mechnikov.

Mechnikov pieced together some of the basic facts about biology and the immune system that we now take so much for granted that it is hard to comprehend that we didn't always know them. He discovered, for example, that white blood cells engulf and destroy bacteria, and he also, in later life, studied the microbiota of the human intestine.

Interestingly, he developed a theory that senility was provoked by poisoning of the body caused by the products of some of our gut bacteria. This theory has not found modern support, although given some of the discoveries being made I wouldn't rule anything out just yet!

To prevent the alleged senility-causing bacteria from thriving, Mechnikov proposed a diet containing milk fermented by lactic acid-producing bacteria. Or, as we might call them, probiotic yogurt drinks.[8]

'Either anally or orally'

Probiotics is a proprietorial approach to gut husbandry that at its most palatable takes the form of those little bottles of 'fancy yogurts'; at the other end of the taste spectrum, we have faecal microbiota transplantation (FMT), also known as stool transplants. Any way you want to dress it up, FMT involves taking someone else's poo into your body more or less (mostly less) processed, thereby introducing beneficial bacteria, either anally or orally. Any medical procedure that ends in the words 'either anally or orally' is probably best put off for as long as possible, so let's start with the fancy yogurts and some other probiotic foodstuffs. Just to be clear, these are designed to be taken orally.

Drinking fancy yogurt doesn't really work

The commercial probiotic market is dominated by 'fermented dairy products', mostly yogurts. These contain various live bacteria that, when ingested, are supposed to confer some benefit over and above that of the basic nutritional value of the yogurt. In other words, we are entering the murky world of commercial products with implied medical advantages. As well as yogurts in handy little bottles for drinking on the go (and for keeping the volume of actual product low and profits high, one suspects), you can find cereal bars to keep you topped up around town, rice cereals for raising those bacterial levels at breakfast and even probiotic dog food for keeping Fido's gut biota bouncing. It is big business, apparently worth £164 million in the UK in 2009,[9] although even that figure pales into insignificance when you consider the global market was estimated to be US$26.1 billion in 2012 and analysts predict further growth.[10] What's even more staggering is that these products don't seem to work.

That's a sweeping and rather bold statement, so I should clarify it. In many cases a probiotic *approach* is beneficial, and clinically based probiotic procedures like FMT, administering probiotics with antibiotics and some other applications have supported and potentially important advantages that I will get to shortly. Drinking expensive yogurt or other commercially available preparations containing bacteria with implied probiotic properties, on the other hand, have very little evidence to support any benefit, at least not for the form in which they are ingested, and not at the moment. This is not to say that they couldn't, or won't in the future but that's the situation now. At the time of writing, the European Food Standards Agency and the US FDA have not approved *any* health claims for these products and 'probiotic' is not a word you will see on a visit to the supermarket in Europe, where it has been effectively banned since the end of 2012.[11]

If you were to put 'probiotic' on food packaging you would absolutely, and without any room for reasonable doubt, be making a health claim. You are not simply saying that the product 'contains bacteria', because firstly such a statement would be trivial and secondly it would be a marketing catastrophe. Many foodstuffs are allowed by law to contain a legal maximum level of insect 'parts' (they are unavoidable when you think about the whole field-to-plate process), but no manufacturer in their right mind is going to state 'contains insects' on the packaging.[12] However, since manufacturers can't make health claims and so can't use 'probiotic', they are left with no option but to talk about the bacteria their product contains and to skate as close to the legal side of the line as they can in describing it. Hence we see the proliferation on food labels of scientific names that would have been unfamiliar and meaningless to most of us ten years ago and yet now trip off the tongue like we've always known them. Reading the labels in the yogurt cabinet aloud these days sounds as if you're giving a benediction: *Lactobacillus casei immunitas, casei Shirota, Bifidus regularis, Bifidus digestivum, Qui vivis et regnas in saecula saeculorum*. Amen to that. There is also a proliferation of the word 'live', as in 'cereal bar with live yogurt', which is clearly more marketable than the alternative. I can't imagine 'dead yogurt bars' shifting too many units.

Given that in many places manufacturers can't use the term probiotic and that this prohibition results from a lack of evidence supporting their implied medical benefits, why is the industry still prospering? I think part of the reason involves, appropriately enough, a symbiotic relationship between the 'probiotic' industry and the media.

Probiotic approaches can and do work

To explain what I mean, we need to examine those situations where the probiotic approach does work. One of the best cases is that of antibiotic-associated diarrhoea (AAD) in children. Antibiotics wipe out the gut bacteria and there is now reasonable, but not bomb-proof, evidence that administering probiotics containing high doses of *Lactobacilli*, *Bifidobacterium*, *Streptococcus* or *Saccharomyces boulardii* (a yeast and therefore a fungus rather than a bacterium) alone or in combination may be effective for preventing, or reducing the effects of, AAD in children. The work is ongoing, though, and much more research is needed to evaluate fully the beneficial effects of probiotics in protecting against AAD.[13]

The key phrase in the preceding paragraph is 'high doses'. The probiotics are medically prepared and administered in a clinical setting. These tests aren't about giving little Sarah a yogurt drink from the local shop in her lunchbox. A related area where the medical use of probiotics has some evidential support is in reducing the risk of developing diarrhoea should you contract a *Clostridium difficile* infection.

Clostridium difficile, or 'C. diff', is a bacterium that often causes issues for people taking antibiotics. Normally, it isn't much of a problem in the gut, but if the gut community is disturbed by the use of antibiotics then it can proliferate and cause diarrhoea, cramps and a high temperature. It can also lead to life-threatening complications including a severe swelling in the colon caused by a build-up of gas. It is common in healthcare settings, which is unsurprising given that they have a relatively high proportion of people taking antibiotics. A number of studies and meta-analyses, which collect and analyse the results of multiple studies, have provided 'moderate' evidence that probiotics are safe and effective for preventing C. *diff*-associated diarrhoea. As with AAD, probiotics are an interesting avenue for therapeutic solutions to a major problem, but the evidence is still being assembled and the probiotics being used are clinically administered in high doses.[14]

Probiotics may also reduce the likelihood of premature babies developing necrotising enterocolitis (a condition where parts of the bowel undergo tissue death, or necrosis)[15], may help with IBS (but which strain of bacteria, how much to ingest and who might benefit is far from clear)[16] and could be effective in lactose intolerance (this is really at the 'give it a go if you want, we're still collecting evidence' stage).[17] One thing the evidence certainly doesn't support, despite claims by the industry, is that probiotics 'boost your immune system'.[18]

It is inevitable that people should be interested in their health and also that 'current' health issues such as the rise in IBS, antibiotic resistance and the possibility of supplementing our gut microbiota with probiotics should attract media attention. Almost any research that suggests any sort of benefit at all seems to get covered. At the time of writing this very sentence (around midday), there are already eight stories about probiotics in the world's media displaying on my Google News search for today. Six of these stories are from news sources within Europe or the US, where the relevant authorities have imposed strict regulation over the use of the term probiotic and have yet to acknowledge any benefit of commercially available products aimed at public consumption. Three of the stories from Europe, where remember you can't put 'probiotic' on products, *feature a photo of a yogurt* despite the research they mention not referring to yogurt in any way!

A photograph of yogurt has become a visual shorthand for 'probiotic', so who cares what the European Food Safety Standards Agency and other agencies say about using the term? When the press creates such a strong connection between probiotics (which are nearly always reported positively) and specific products, the labelling regulations are largely irrelevant. The message the manufacturers would like to broadcast is that their 'fermented dairy products' are 'probiotic' and therefore bring a 'health benefit'. They can't give this message out because there is *no evidence for such a claim* for these products, at least at the moment. Fortunately, they can obey the regulations to the letter while the press continues to cover 'probiotics' favourably and directly associate credible medical evidence concerning clinical interventions with what amount to little more than overpriced drinkable yogurts, albeit with some bacterial 'contamination' thrown in. I wish I'd thought of it.

What about 'the other end'?

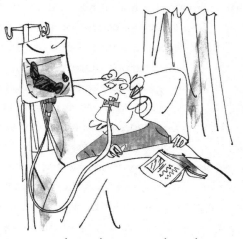

Consuming gut microbiota bacteria cultured in yogurt or some other foodstuff is one way to get them into your system, but it has clear issues. Firstly, we know that the bacteria in the gut make a complex multi-species and multi-strain community with differences between different gut regions, but 'probiotic' products inevitably lack this biodiversity. Secondly, bacteria taken orally but destined for the more anal end of the gut (like the colon) have to survive a pretty challenging journey to make it to their intended destination. Given that poo contains a high number and good diversity of bacteria generally reflective of the gut community and that the anus is closer to bacterially rich parts of the gut than the mouth, it is not hard to devise potentially more effective ways to achieve a change in the gut microbiota (which is the point of a probiotic approach) than taking cultured probiotics. You could ingest some poo, or, even better, you could shove some up your backside.

Using a refreshingly simple technique, faecal microbiota transplantation (FMT) takes poo from a donor, processes it slightly and inserts it into the gut of a recipient. As the UK National Institute for Health and Care Excellence (NICE) put it, 'Donor faeces are taken and diluted with water, saline or another liquid such as milk or yogurt, and subsequently strained to remove large particles.[19] The resulting suspension is introduced into the recipient's gut via a nasogastric tube, nasoduodenal tube, rectal enema or via the biopsy channel of a colonoscope.' In other words, someone else's strained poo, and their microbiota, get into your gut through either the front or the back door.

FMT really does work, but at the moment its use is mostly limited to patients with recurrent *Clostridium difficile* infections. The crucial words here seem to be 'at the moment', since this is a fast-moving area with buckets of potential for new therapeutic opportunities.[20] In *C. diff* cases, the evidence points to FMT being something of a wonder therapy: medical papers talk of 90% of patients suffering from recurrent *C. diff* infection being cured by it.[21] Given that *C. diff* infection (CDI) is increasing and can be fatal, FMT offers a treatment that is safe, effective and a lot cheaper and more sensible than continued antibiotic assault. Initial scepticism has been replaced by papers that outline the case for making FMT the 'go to' treatment for recurrent CDI, and suggesting protocols and procedures for administering it.

An obvious next step is to consider FMT as a therapeutic option for people with IBD, and this potential has generated considerable enthusiasm with many researchers examining FMT as a treatment for ulcerative colitis and Crohn's disease. There are some intriguing case studies suggesting some success with both, but moving from case studies to a convincing evidence base and subsequent therapy requires properly defined and executed trials on large numbers of patients, something we currently lack.[22]

We now know just how important our gut microbiota is in diseases that initially seem unrelated to the microscopic single-celled bacteria dwelling within our intestines. This knowledge inevitably makes FMT, if not a therapeutic solution right now, then a clear candidate for some serious investigation in a surprisingly wide range of diseases. As well as treatment for IBD, scientists are already considering FMT as a potential (and note the guarded language) therapeutic option worthy of investigation for IBS, metabolic syndrome (having the dangerous triumvirate of diabetes, obesity and high blood pressure that affects as many as one in four adults in the UK), autoimmune diseases and allergies.[23]

We saw in Chapter Eight that transferring microbes from an obese person to a germfree mouse resulted in obese mice and that microbial communities associated with leanness could be used as a therapy for obesity – in association with diet and exercise, of course. This is a probiotic approach, reseeding your internal lawn and, as with worrying about your lawn, you could be forgiven for thinking that microbial treatments are 'first world' solutions to 'first world' problems. However, that need not be the case in the long term.

Kwashiorkor is a form of malnutrition that affects a lot of people in the developing world. It causes many symptoms and is not yet fully understood. Perhaps the most immediately recognisable symptom is the 'pot belly' seen all too often on children in areas where sustained nutrition is hard to come by. In a study on twins in Malawi, researchers transplanted microbes from children with kwashiorkor into germfree mice and were able to transfer that malnutrition to the recipient mice. Remarkably, mice that received microbes from identical twins of sick children who did not have kwashiorkor did not develop malnutrition. Research continues, but now the goal is to move away from germfree mice. Alternatives are expensive and far from straightforward, but a test-tube-based system and ultimately a computer-modelling approach based on DNA sequences will one day provide inexpensive insights into the bacterial connection with diseases and potential therapeutic options that already seem tantalisingly close.[24]

CHAPTER ELEVEN

The Captain's Log: Final Thoughts...

We've come a very long way since we sat on the toilet back in Chapter One and thought about our poo, although with faecal microbiota transplants fresh in our minds you could argue that we've got back to where we started. It's certainly been a revealing round trip, taking in our bathrooms, kitchens, hand hygiene (and the lack of it), the food we eat, the drugs we use and abuse, our hidden inner jungle, our immune system, mental health, obesity, allergies and more than a little bacterial biology along the way.

Bacteria have an enormous influence in our lives. In fact, without them we really aren't 'us' at all. Within virtually every cell in our bodies are tiny structures called mitochondria where the chemical processes of respiration occur and these minute structures were, back in the primordial soup, free-living bacteria. At some point, a truly momentous point in the evolution of life, a bigger cell engulfed them and, rather than consuming them, those cells began an intimate partnership that led to the plants, animals, fungi and all the large-scale life and complexity we see all around us. Partnerships and relationships also exist with the bacteria that live within and on our bodies, and their interactions with us and our health are complex. As we've seen, understanding those interactions requires us to understand our bodies not as 'ours' but as complex entangled ecosystems. That's quite a leap.

The problem we all face is that while science is untangling our complex relationships with bacteria, we are subjected to a constant drip-feed of information and interpretation, theory and counter-theory through an ever-excitable media. An obsession with health and a scientific community keen to gain coverage of new research mean that, more than ever before, scientifically complex information is pushed onto a public that doesn't always have the knowledge to appreciate the limitations and implications of what they are reading. It's not just a problem for the public; I know plenty of professional scientists who sometimes feel as if they are drowning in new findings and published papers, endlessly spurting from the information hoses of Twitter, Facebook and email.

Before the electronic information age, science largely happened behind closed doors. As ideas developed and evidence was gathered, a consensus was allowed to form and, given enough time, that consensus would make it out of the 'club' and into the wider world. In those days, as now, science was not filled with newsworthy 'Eureka!' moments but was instead a rather slow and laborious process where each small and not especially important finding added to the last, building up a consensus brick by brick and largely hidden from view. By the time Joe Public got to see it, the 'house' was built. Sure, science might add a few extra windows and doors here and there as new findings were made, but the overall structure was clearly defined and well supported.

This new world of readily available science is genuinely exciting, not least because we all get to see the 'house' being built. The problem is that we inevitably like to imagine what it will look like and, reading media stories covering gut bacteria and IBD, IBS, allergies and obesity, or the virtues of prebiotics, probiotics and faecal transplants, you'd be forgiven for thinking that it had already been built. However, while journalists are speculating on

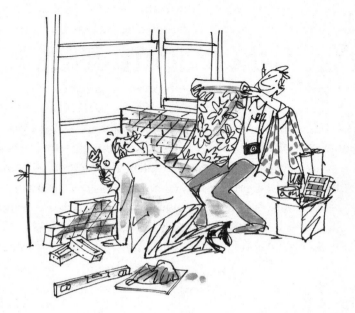

the colour of the attic carpet, scientists are often still digging the foundations. One thing is absolutely certain, though: bacteria are going to be a major partner in our medical future. Worth thinking about the next time you flush the toilet ...

Acknowledgements

This book would not have been written if the BBC Radio Science Unit hadn't taken me under their wing and at some point along the way let me present a documentary about gut bacteria. My thanks to all the wonderful people there that I've had the pleasure to work with. In the face of ever deeper budget cuts they continue to make scientific documentaries of the very highest quality for BBC Radio 4 and the BBC World Service. Long may they continue to do so.

Notes and references

The notes and references in the text are explained below. Wherever possible, I have chosen sources that are freely available online. Scholar.Google.com is a very useful free-to-use site for locating scientific papers, and searching for authors and titles often yields PDFs of papers that might otherwise be unobtainable outside of a university or hospital library.

Chapter 1: Are You Sitting Comfortably?

1. This study was widely reported in 2001. A more straight-faced account can be found on the BBC's news site under the heading 'Millions read on the toilet', published 20 March 2001 and available at http://news.bbc.co.uk/1/hi/health/1230115.stm.

2. The number of bacteria on Earth was estimated by William Whitman and colleagues in a paper published in 1998 in the *Proceedings of the National Academy of Sciences of the United States of America* (usually abbreviated to PNAS). It's an interesting read and a great example of how to make a scientifically credible estimate of a seemingly ungraspable number. The full reference is Whitman et al. 1998 'Prokaryotes: the unseen majority'. *PNAS* 95: 6578–6583.

3. There are numerous studies estimating oral bacteria diversity and the problem of defining a bacterial species (which is discussed in Chapter Two) can make these estimates complicated. In a sense, the actual number is less important than the take-home message, which is that bacteria in the mouth are remarkably diverse! However, the figure of 700–750 species is widely used in the literature and is discussed on the Human Oral Microbiome Database http://

www.homd.org/. The higher figures are discussed in Keijser et al. 2008 Pyrosequencing analysis of the oral microflora of healthy adults. *Journal of Dental Research* 87:1016–1020 and in Zaura et al. 2009 Defining the healthy 'core microbiome' of oral microbial communities. *BMC Microbiology* 9: 259.

4. The problems of growing unculturable bacteria are discussed in Stewart 2012 'Growing unculturable bacteria'. *Journal of Bacteriology* 194: 4151--4160. An exciting recent advance in culturing soil bacteria is the iChip, which cultures bacteria in tiny holes in a small rectangular 'plate' enclosed by semi-permeable membranes. This technology resulted in a paper that attracted considerable attention at the start of 2015: Ling et al. 2015 'A new antibiotic kills pathogens without detectable resistance.' *Nature* 517: 455-459. The iChip can be seen at www.bbc.co.uk/news/health-30657486.

5. The bacterial diversity associated with tooth decay is considered in Chhour [sic] et al. 2005 'Molecular analysis of microbial diversity in advanced caries.' *Journal of Clinical Microbiology* 43: 843–849.

6. Howard Jenkinson and Richard Lamont provide an interesting overview of 'Oral microbial communities in sickness and in health' in their paper with this title in *Trends in Microbiology* 2005 13: 589–595.

7. There are many sites and organisations devoted to inflammatory bowel diseases. For a good, medical overview of symptoms see http://www.nhs.uk/conditions/Inflammatory-bowel-disease/Pages/Introduction.aspx. Beware of internet-hypochondria and self-diagnosis! If you think you are ill, you should see a doctor, not an internet browser...

8. The latest figures on the global epidemic of HIV and AIDS can be found at www.avert.org and linked pages. It is a sobering read.

9. Ben Goldacre's excellent book *Bad Science* provides all you could want to know about the representation, use and abuse of statistics in medicine and other areas of life. His website http://www.badscience.net/ is always an entertaining browse.

10. For a useful timeline of the development of ADHD as a diagnosis,

its treatment and its prevalence, see www.cdc.gov/ncbddd/adhd/documents/timeline.pdf published by the United States' Centers for Disease Control and Prevention.

11. The reality of the rise of inflammatory bowel diseases, an overview of their occurrence and factors related to their rise are reviewed in Loftus Jr 2004 Clinical epidemiology of inflammatory bowel disease: Incidence, prevalence, and environmental influences. *Gastroenterology* 126: 1504–1517. A global overview is provided by Economou and Pappas 2008 New global map of Crohn's disease: Genetic, environmental, and socioeconomic correlations. *Inflammatory Bowel Disease* 14: 709–720.

12. For an upbeat overview of this new frontier of medical science, read David Grogan's introductory comments to a *Nature Innovations in the Microbiome* special (http://www.nature.com/nature/journal/v518/n7540_supp/full/518S2a.html). In this short article, entitled 'The Microbes Within', Grogan states that 'Revelations about the role of the human microbiome in our lives have begun to shake the foundations of medicine and nutrition'. Indeed they have, as we'll see ...

Chapter 2: 'Kills 99% of known germs'

1. For a very readable review of the rise of the cane toad in Australia and attempts to control it, it is worth exploring the Biodiversity and Invasive Species sections of the Australian Government Department of the Environment's website. The cane toad section is currently at www.environment.gov.au/biodiversity/invasive-species/feral-animals-australia/cane-toads.

2. Other risk factors for UTIs include the age at which you first contract a UTI and the UTI history of your mother. You can read more about it in Scholes et al. (2000) Risk factors for recurrent urinary tract infection in young women. *The Journal of Infectious Diseases* 182: 1177–1182.

3. *E. coli* as a prominent cause of UTI infections is discussed in

Zhang and Foxman 2003 Molecular epidemiology of *Escherichia coli* mediated urinary tract infections. *Frontiers in Bioscience* 1;8:e235–44, available at https://www.bioscience.org/2003/v8/e/1007/fulltext. htm.

4. The potential for toilet flushing to cause contamination is explored in Barker and Jones 2005 'The potential spread of infection caused by aerosol contamination of surfaces after flushing a domestic toilet.' *Journal of Applied Microbiology* 99: 339–347. The value of having a toilet lid, and of keeping it shut when flushing, was shown by Best et al 2012 Potential for aerosolization of *Clostridium difficile* after flushing toilets: the role of toilet lids in reducing environmental contamination risk. *Journal of Hospital Infection* 80: 1–5.

5. This sage advice, rarely followed in my experience, can be found at http://www.nhs.uk/Livewell/homehygiene/Pages/food-and-home-hygiene-facts.aspx.

6. The potential perils of poo for contact-lens wearers are discussed in Hall and Jones 2010 Contact Lens cases: the missing link in contact-lens safety. *Eye and Contact Lens* 36: 101–105.

7. For some insight into the weird world of *E. coli* taxonomy, including the conclusion that there is likely a 'continuum rather than sharp species borders in this group' (hardly making the 'species concept' any simpler!) see Lukjancenko et al 2010 Comparison of 61 sequenced *Escherichia coli* genomes.' *Microbial Ecology* 60: 708–720.

8. The role of beef in the transmission of O157:H7 is discussed in Armstrong et al. 1996 Emerging foodborne pathogens: *Escherichia coli* O157:H7 as a model of entry of a new pathogen into the food supply of the developed world. *Epidemiologic Reviews* 18: 29–51.

9. For some interesting reading on 20 years of outbreaks of O157:H7 in the United States, have a look at Rangel et al. 2005 Epidemiology of *Escherichia coli* O157:H7 outbreaks, United States, 1982–2002 *Emerging Infectious Diseases* 11: 603–609.

10. For a reasonably readable introduction to Shiga toxins and their mode of action, try Sandvig 2001 Shiga toxins *Toxicon* 39: 1629–1635.

11. The World Health Organization's European Office tracks this outbreak and in some cases traces it to specific sources as well as offering advice www.euro.who.int/en/health-topics/emergencies/international-health-regulations/outbreaks-of-e.-coli-o104h4-infection.

12. The role played by phages and an interesting antibiotic angle are both discussed in *Phage on the Rampage* www.nature.com/news/2011/110609/full/news.2011.360.html.

13. If you wish to scare yourself about the state of your toothbrush bristles, then check out Ferreira et al. 2012 Microbiological evaluation of bristles of frequently used toothbrushes. *Dental Press Journal of Orthodontics* 17: 72–76. Just remember, 'presence' does not always mean 'actual problem'.

14. The persistence of *Salmonella* is examined by Barker and Bloomfield 2000 Survival of *Salmonella* in bathrooms and toilets in domestic homes following salmonellosis. *Journal of Applied Microbiology* 89: 137–144.

15. How household bleach kills bacteria is described in an article of the same name published by *Science Daily* using sources from the University of Michigan http://www.sciencedaily.com/releases/2008/11/081113140314.htm.

16. The story of HSP33, and some more information on the action of bleach, is revealed in the very readable article 'How does bleach bleach?' by Heidi Ledford at http://www.nature.com/news/2008/081113/full/news.2008.1228.html.

17. The use of ATP to monitor cleaning and the effectiveness, or otherwise, of hospital cleaning practices are studied by Boyce et al. Monitoring the effectiveness of hospital cleaning practices by use of an adenosine triphosphate bioluminescence assay. *Infection Control and Hospital Epidemiology* 30: 678–684.

18. The effectiveness of acetic acid against mycobacteria, specifically *Mycobacterium tuberculosis*, is shown by Cortesia et al. 2014 Acetic acid, the active component of vinegar, is an effective tuberculocidal disinfectant. *mBio* 5: e00013–14.

19. You can view the statistics of *Shigella* cases in the UK at https://www.gov.uk/government/collections/shigella-guidance-data-and-analysis ...

20. ...and *Salmonella* can viewed at https://www.gov.uk/government/uploads/system/uploads/attachment_data/file/337647/Salmonella_surveillance_tables.pdf.

21. The Illinois Poison Center has a wonderful section entitled 'My Child Ate...' with a list that demonstrates the powerful omnivory of the young human. The section is at http://illinoispoisoncenter.org/my-child-ate and the section on poo can be found at http://illinoispoisoncenter.org/my-child-ate-poop. It contains the useful observation that 'The most common feces ingested by children include human (their own), cat, dog and bird'.

Chapter 3: If you can't stand the heat ...

1. This ridiculously precise figure is widely reported, along with other equally precise values, and can usually be traced back to the Hygiene Council. This 'council' is funded by Reckitt Benckiser, the company that makes Lysol-branded cleaning and disinfecting products. You can explore your home via their interactive website at www.hygienecouncil.org/. Just bear in mind ... this is a company that wants to sell you products for killing bacteria. I'm just saying...

2. More bacteria paranoia, this time fuelled by the UK's *Daily Mail* newspaper in 2012: The kitchen sponge is 200,000 times dirtier than a toilet seat – and could even lead to PARALYSIS [the capitals appear in the headline – just to be sure that you get THE MESSAGE!] www.dailymail.co.uk/health/article-2235650/The-kitchen-sponge-200-000-times-dirtier-toilet-seat--lead-PARALYSIS.html#ixzz3SZ7yIBMw.

3. For the low-down on *Listeria* in the home, read Beumer et al. 1996 *Listeria* species in domestic environments. *Epidemiology and Infection* 117: 437–442.

4. Facts and figures about listeriosis in the US are readily available

at www.cdc.gov/listeria/statistics.html and links from this site.

5. Reported faecal carriage rates of *Listeria monocytogenes* (i.e. listeriosis-causing bacteria in poo) in all sorts of people are detailed by Slutsker and Schuchat 1999 Listeriosis in humans. In *Listeria, Listeriosis and Food Safety* edited by Ryser and Marth (Chapter 4, 75–95). New York, Basel: Marcel Dekker, Inc.

6. Details of how *Listeria* causes listeriosis can be found in *Todar's Online Textbook of Bacteriology* by Kenneth Todar textbookofbacteriology. net/Listeria_1.html and linked pages.

7. The Jensen Farm outbreak is reported by the Centers for Disease Control and Prevention in their Morbidity and Mortality Weekly Report (MMWR) of 7 October 2011: Multistate Outbreak of Listeriosis Associated with Jensen Farms Cantaloupe, United States, August–September 2011. MMWR 60: 1357–1358. The avoidance of jail is reported widely in the US media, for example by Mary Beth Marklein in *USA Today* on 28 January 2014: Cantaloupe farmers get no prison time in disease outbreak www.usatoday.com/story/ news/nation/2014/01/28/sentencing-of-colorado-cantaloupe-farmers/4958671/.

8. Information on how *Salmonella* infects us, and a rather neat animation of the process, can be found at *Intracellular Infection by Salmonella* published by the Howard Hughes Medical Institute www.hhmi. org/biointeractive/intracellular-infection-salmonella.

9. This figure is reported by the US Food and Drug Administration at www.fda.gov/Food/ResourcesForYou/Consumers/ucm077342. htm. The site also contains a wealth of information on *Salmonella* and how to avoid it.

10. This outbreak was covered by a number of news sources in the UK, for example in *The Guardian* (and links within this article) www. theguardian.com/society/2014/aug/15/salmonella-outbreak-england-investigation.

11. Widely covered in the UK's media, for example by David Millward in the *Daily Telegraph* www.telegraph.co.uk/news/uknews/1366276/ Currie-was-right-on-salmonella.html.

12. Public Health Wales provides some interesting facts and figures, as well as confirming the importance of compulsory vaccination of the UK's egg-laying flock at www.wales.nhs.uk/sites3/page. cfm?orgid=457&pid=48023.

13. The Street Spice Festival outbreak is outlined at www.newcastle. gov.uk/news-story/street-spice-festival-outbreak-investigation-concludes and is detailed in the Public Health England report available here: www.newcastle.gov.uk/sites/drupalncc.newcastle.gov.uk/files/wwwfileroot/environment/environmental_health/20130617_ street_spice_oct_report_-_final.pdf.

14. The ever-useful Centers for Disease Control and Prevention in the US has an overview of the occurrence of *Salmonella* in reptiles, and the legal situation at www.cdc.gov/features/salmonellafrogturtle/ and links therein. If you really can't wait to read the Federal Code then you can find it here: www.accessdata.fda.gov/scripts/cdrh/ cfdocs/cfcfr/CFRSearch.cfm?fr=1240.62.

15. The full list can be located at www.cdc.gov/ecoli/outbreaks.html.

16. The full list of cases recorded in England and Wales between 2000 and 2012 can be viewed at https://www.gov.uk/government/ publications/campylobacter-cases-2000-to-2012.

17. An overview of the symptoms and treatment of this condition can be found at http://www.nhs.uk/conditions/Guillain-Barre-syndrome/Pages/Introduction.aspx.

18. The review of the link between *Campylobacter* and Guillain-Barré Syndrome mentioned in this section was undertaken in Poropatich et al. 2010 Quantifying the association between *Campylobacter* infection and Guillain-Barré Syndrome: A systematic review. *Journal of Health, Population and Nutrition* 28: 454–552.

19. *Campylobacter* and gastroenteritis, including incidences and general information, are surveyed in a highly readable paper by Galanis 2007 *Campylobacter* and gastroenteritis. *Canadian Medical Association Journal* 177: 570–571.

20. The presence of *Campylobacter* in starling poo is described by Colles et al. 2009 Dynamics of *Campylobacter* colonization of a natural host,

Sturnus vulgaris (European Starling). *Environmental Microbiology* 11: 258–267.

21. A summary of this report and some sensible advice is published at www.food.gov.uk/news-updates/news/2014/9279/campylobacter-survey.

22. You know it makes sense . . . http://www.cdc.gov/healthywater/swimming/rwi/rwi-prevent.html.

23. The Centers for Disease Control and Prevention's advice on vegetables can be found at http://www.cdc.gov/nutrition/everyone/fruitsvegetables/foodsafety.html and the UK's National Health Service's advice is at http://www.nhs.uk/Livewell/homehygiene/Pages/How-to-wash-fruit-and-vegetables.aspx. Worth following . . .

Chapter 4: Why you should think twice about shaking hands (especially with men)

1. A value of 1.1 million lives a year (lower estimate 0.5 million, upper estimate 1.4 million) is calculated in a systematic review of studies linking diarrhoeal deaths and hand-washing by Curtis and Cairncross 2003 Effect of washing hands with soap on diarrhoea risk in the community: a systematic review. *The Lancet Infectious Diseases* 3: 275–281.

2. Ultra-violet disclosure hand-washing kits are widely and cheaply available online, as are UV LED torches. It's a nice way to teach children, plus you can use the UV torch to pretend you're in *CSI*.

3. There are plenty of hand-hygiene sites offering advice on what to do, and in some cases (see the Centers for Disease Control and Prevention references further down) offering scientific studies supporting the suggested procedure. In terms of easy-to-follow advice, though www.wash-hands.com/hand_hygiene_and_you/how_to_wash_your_hands is simple, clear and effective.

4. This study was undertaken by Johnson et al. 2003 Sex differences in public restroom handwashing behaviour associated with visual behaviour prompts. *Perceptual and Motor Skills* 97: 805–810.

5. These and other data can be found in Borchgrevink et al. 2013 Hand washing practices in a college town environment. *Journal of Environmental Health* 75: 18–24.

6. There are many hand-hygiene studies out there and they are often reported in the popular press. The numbers differ but the overall message doesn't. We don't wash our hands very reliably, very well or for very long. Monk-Turner et al 2005 Another look at hand washing behavior. *Social Behavior and Personality: an international journal* 33: 629–634 is as good a summary as any, finding that women wash hands more often than men and that very few wash for anywhere near long enough.

7. The US Centers for Disease Control and Prevention has a fantastic website that details the scientific evidence behind correct hand hygiene, as well as links to the studies themselves. It can be accessed at www.cdc.gov/handwashing/show-me-the-science-handwashing.html.

8. This is covered by the same study as in note 4.

9. A rather sobering study for those of us lucky enough to have fresh, clean, running water, this research is reported in Luby et al. 2001 Microbiologic effectiveness of hand washing with soap in an urban squatter settlement, Karachi, Pakistan. *Epidemiology and Infection* 127: 237–244.

10. The CDC's website detailed in note 7 covers this point, as do Michaels et al. 2002 Water temperature as a factor in handwashing efficacy. *Food Service Technology* 2: 139–149.

11. The ever-useful CDC website 'Show me the Science' again provides an excellent source of *bona fide* studies examining aspects of hand hygiene. www.cdc.gov/handwashing/show-me-the-science-handwashing.html.

12. The value of scrubbing is demonstrated by Burton et al. 2011 The effect of handwashing with water or soap on bacterial contamination of hands. *International Journal of Environmental Research and Public Health* 8: 97–104.

13. A great review of hand-drying techniques is provided by Huang et

al. 2012 The hygienic efficacy of different hand-drying methods: A review of the evidence. *Mayo Clinic Proceedings* 87: 791–798.

14. This point is covered in Huang et al. 2012, note 13 above.

15. This glorious headline appeared in 2009 and can be found at news. bbc.co.uk/1/hi/england/dorset/8272799.stm.

16. The value of alcohol gels for reducing skin dryness and irritation in those washing their hands frequently has been studied by Boyce et al. 2000 Skin irritation and dryness associated with two hand-hygiene regimens: soap-and-water hand washing versus hand antisepsis with an alcoholic hand gel. *Infection Control and Hospital Epidemiology* 21: 442–448.

17. A treasure-trove of scientific studies on sanitisers and hand gels can be found by following the links at www.cdc.gov/handwashing/show-me-the-science-hand-sanitizer.html.

18. The link between hand sanitisers and reduced absenteeism was investigated in Dyer et al. 2000 Alcohol-free instant hand sanitizer reduces elementary school illness absenteeism. *Family Medicine* 32: 633–638.

19. For an updated situation report on the US FDA's position visit www. fda.gov/forconsumers/consumerupdates/ and search for 'triclosan'.

20. Tracking down information on EU bans, and distinguishing 'calls for a ban' and 'proposals for a ban' from 'a ban' is not as easy as it should be. However, for some EU-related information, look at ec.europa. eu/health/scientific_committees/opinions_layman/triclosan/en/l-3/2-uses-cosmetics-disinfectant.htm#4p0 and, for its ban on certain product types, see eur-lex.europa.eu/legal-content/EN/TXT/PDF/?uri=CELEX:32014D0227&from=EN.

21. For a review of triclosan and resistance, look at Yazdankhah et al. 2006 Triclosan and antimicrobial resistance in bacteria: an overview. *Microbial Drug Resistance* 12: 83–90; and more recently Bedoux et al. 2012 Occurrence and toxicity of antimicrobial triclosan and by-products in the environment. *Environmental Science and Pollution Research International* 19: 1044–1065, which concludes that 'the excessive use of TCS [*5-chloro-2,4-dichlorophenoxyphenol, or triclosan*]

is suspected to increase the risk of emergence of TCS-resistant bacteria and the selection of resistant strains'.

Chapter 5: Resistance is not useless

1. The decrease in salmonellosis in the UK as a consequence of vaccinating poultry is discussed by O'Brien 2013 The 'decline and fall' of nontyphoidal *Salmonella* in the United Kingdom. *Clinical Infectious Diseases* 56: 705–710.

2. An example of one approach being taken is provided by Layton et al 2011 Evaluation of *Salmonella*-vectored Campylobacter peptide epitopes for reduction of *Campylobacter jejuni* in broiler chickens. *Clinical and Vaccine Immunology* 18: 449–454.

3. The EU ban, and the sequence of antibiotics banned from 1997, are discussed in a useful book chapter entitled 'Antibiotic resistance: linking human and animal health' by Henrik Wegener appearing as Chapter A15, pp331–349 in *Improving Food Safety Through a One Health Approach: Workshop Summary* published by The National Academies Press, USA.

4. The FDA's approach is explained in a 2012 news release of theirs entitled *FDA takes steps to protect public health* and is available at www.fda.gov/NewsEvents/Newsroom/PressAnnouncements/ ucm299802.htm.

5. To read more about the UK government's position on antibiotic resistance, visit www.gov.uk/government/news/prime-minister-warns-of-global-threat-of-antibiotic-resistance.

6. The World Health Organization's (WHO) report is called *Antimicrobial resistance: global report on surveillance 2014* and is available at www.who.int/drugresistance/documents/ surveillancereport/en/. It's a scary read.

7. This refers to the WHO report *Antimicrobial resistance: global report on surveillance 2014* detailed in note 6.

8. For some good general information on the medical implications of *Staphylococcus aureus* infection, read Naber 2009 *Staphylococcus*

aureus bacteremia: epidemiology, pathophysiology, and management strategies. *Clinical Infectious Diseases* 48 (Supplement 4) S213–S237.

9. Nasal carriage is explored by Kluytmans et al. 1997 Nasal carriage of *Staphylococcus aureus*: epidemiology, underlying mechanisms, and associated risks. *Clinical Microbiology Reviews* 10: 505–520.

10. For a primer in antibiotic resistance including information on beta-lactamases, which break down penicillin, visit *Todar's Online Textbook of Bacteriology* at http://textbookofbacteriology.net/resantimicrobial.html.

11. An excellent article charting the rise of penicillin resistance in *Staphylococcus aureus* is Chambers 2001 The Changing Epidemiology of *Staphylococcus aureus? Emerging Infectious Diseases* 7: March–April, available at http://wwwnc.cdc.gov/eid/article/7/2/70-0178_article.

12. For more information on plasmids and resistance, take a look at Bennett 2008 Plasmid encoded antibiotic resistance: acquisition and transfer of antibiotic resistance genes in bacteria. *British Journal of Pharmacology* 153(Supplement 1): S347–S357.

13. Further information on bacterial genetics can be found at www.biologyreference.com/Ar-Bi/Bacterial-Genetics.html or in most general biology textbooks.

14. This review is Phillips et al. Does the use of antibiotics in food animals pose a risk to human health? A critical review of published data. *Journal of Antimicrobial Chemotherapy* 53: 28–52.

15. The two sides of this argument are debated in a 'Head to Head' article in the *British Medical Journal* (2013, 347: f4214) entitled 'Does adding routine antibiotics to animal feed pose a serious risk to human health?' This article pits David Wallinga against David G S Burch. Wallinga says a ban is possible without damaging food productivity, but Burch argues that the drugs used in agriculture are not those causing problems with resistance in humans.

16. Marshall and Levy 2011 Food animals and antimicrobials: impacts on human health. *Clinical Microbiology Reviews* 24: 718–733.

17. For more about the iChip, see note 4 in Chapter One above.

18. This research is described and discussed in 'Cave bacteria could help develop future antibiotics', published in 2012 and available at www.bbc.co.uk/news/health-19520629.

19. The potential power of nanoscale explosions is discussed in an understandable way in the article 'Buckybomb shows potential power of nanoscale explosives' available at phys.org/news/2015-03-buckybomb-potential-power-nanoscale-explosives.html. The original research paper is Chaban et al. 2015 Buckybomb: Reactive Molecular Dynamics Simulation. *The Journal of Physical Chemistry Letters* 6: 913–917.

20. The potential for buckybombs to target bacteria is discussed in 'Buckybombs could battle bacteria', published in *New Scientist* 223: Issue 2985, p16.

Chapter 6: The world within

1. This wonderful estimate comes from Bianconi et al. 2013 An estimation of the number of cells in the human body. *Annals of Human Biology* 40: 463–471.

2. There are many estimates out there but the lower numbers cited appear in Qiin et al. 2013 A human gut microbial gene catalog established by metagenomic sequencing. *Nature* 464: 59–65. They suggest that we harbour 'between 1000 and 1150 prevalent bacterial species and each individual at least 160 such species, which are also largely shared'. The value of 1000 '"species-level" phylotypes: clusters of sequences that have as much diversity . . . as named species' is cited in Lozupone et al. 2012 Diversity, stability and resilience of the human gut microbiota. *Nature* 489: 220–230. The latter is a very readable article that is available free online and worth tracking down: try http://www.ncbi.nlm.nih.gov/pmc/articles/PMC3577372/. Other numbers for the diversity sit somewhere in the middle: 300–500, for example, is cited in Guarner and Malagelada 2003 Gut flora in health and disease. *The Lancet* 361: 512–519, also mentioned in note 7 below.

3. *Helicobacter pylori* and its medical significance are explained at www. patient.co.uk/health/helicobacter-pylori-and-stomach-pain.

4. An interview with Barry Marshall, in which he describes his work and the fateful moment where he drinks some *Helicobacter pylori* ('Well, here it goes, down the hatch'), can be read and viewed at www.achievement.org/autodoc/printmember/mar1int-1.

5. A review of whether *Helicobacter pylori* should be eradicated or preserved, a discussion of the argument between 'treaters' and 'commensalists' and a host of interesting facts about the bacteria and its medical significance can be read in Sachs and Scott 2012 *Helicobacter pylori*: Eradication or Preservation. *F100 Medicine* 4: 7.

6. Some additional information on the role of bacteria in our nutrition can be found in the article 'Exploring the role of gut bacteria in nutrition' by Jo Napolitano, available at http://www.anl.gov/articles/exploring-role-gut-bacteria-digestion.

7. The proliferation of research in this area makes it very difficult both to keep on top of developments and to find genuinely useful reviews that synthesise what we know into something manageable. An excellent review of gut microbiota and their role in nutrition is Sears 2005 A dynamic partnership: celebrating our gut flora. *Anaerobe* 11: 247–251. Another good read is Guarner and Malagelada 2003 Gut flora in health and disease. *The Lancet* 361: 512–519.

8. Information about 'Intestinal flora and endogenous vitamin synthesis' can be found in the paper of the same name by Hill, published in 1997 in the *European Journal of Cancer Prevention* 6: supplement 1 S43–45. Information on K2 and coagulation is provided by Conly and Stein 1992 The production of menaquinones (vitamin K2) by intestinal bacteria and their role in maintaining coagulation homeostasis. *Progress in Food and Nutrition Science* 16: 307–43.

9. The review mentioned in note 7 above is an excellent place to read up more about the varied role of bacteria in our nutrition: Sears 2005 A dynamic partnership: celebrating our gut flora. *Anaerobe* 11: 247–251.

10. This is explored in a paper with a title that pretty much says it all: Rieger et al. 1999 A diet high in fat and meat but low in dietary fibre increases the genotoxic potential of 'faecal water'. *Carcinogenesis* 20: 2311–2316.

11. Guarner and Malagelada 2003 Gut flora in health and disease. *The Lancet* 361: 512–519 is again an approachable and useful read here.

12. P values and the related concept of confidence intervals can be useful to know a bit more about. A tutorial to get you started can be found at www.students4bestevidence.net/a-beginners-guide-to-interpreting-odds-ratios-confidence-intervals-and-p-values-the-nuts-and-bolts-20-minute-tutorial/.

13. The fact that even identical twins have different gut microbiota profiles is explored by Turnbaugh et al. 2009 A core gut microbiome in obese and lean twins. *Nature* 457: 480–484.

14. This point is made by many authors, but the paper by Turnbaugh et al. cited in note 13 mentions it explicitly, stating that '… it appears that a core gut microbiome exists at the level of metabolic functions. This … supports an ecological view of each individual as an "island" inhabited by unique collections of microbial phylotypes: as in actual islands, different species assemblages converge on shared core functions provided by distinctive components.'

15. We'll return to some therapeutic options in later chapters, but the general idea is covered by Foxx-Orenstein and Chey 2012 Manipulation of the gut microbiota as a novel treatment strategy for gastrointestinal disorders. *The American Journal of Gastroenterology Supplements* 1: 41–46 and by Sekirov et al. 2010 Gut microbiota in health and disease. *Physiological Reviews* 90: 859–904.

Chapter 7: Back to immunity school

1. The importance of toll-like receptors and other details are revealed in Round et al. 2011 The toll-like receptor pathway establishes commensal gut colonization. *Science* 332: 974–977.

2. The importance of gut microbiota in future medicine is discussed by

Grogan 2015 The microbes within. Innovations in the microbiome *Nature*: 518 S2 and by other articles in this special supplement issue.

3. This research can be read in Ivanov et al. 2008 Specific microbiota direct the differentiation of Th17 cells in the mucosa of the small intestine. *Cell Host & Microbe* 4: 337–349.

4. For an excellent overview of the role of gut microbiota in our adaptive immune system, take a look at Lee and Mazmanian 2010 Has the microbiota played a critical role in the evolution of the adaptive immune system? *Science* 330: 1768–1773.

5. The metaphor of a house, a fireplace and burning embers can be found in the concluding remarks of Spasova and Surh 2014 Blowing on Embers: commensal microbiota and our immune system. *Frontiers in Immunology* 5: 318.

6. For some accessible information on IBD try www.crohnsandcolitis. org.uk, www.nhs.uk/Conditions/Crohns-disease/Pages/Causes. aspx and www.mayoclinic.org/diseases-conditions/ulcerative-colitis/basics/causes/con-20043763.

7. Research examining the genetics of IBD and the importance of gut microbes was carried out by Jostin et al. 2012 Host-microbe interactions have shaped the genetic architecture of inflammatory bowel disease. *Nature* 491: 119–124. A readable account of this research can be found at www.sanger.ac.uk/about/press/2012/121031.html.

8. The strong family connection to developing IBD is a consistent finding of research in this area. An accessible and often cited work discussing this is Russell and Satsangi 2004 IBD: a family affair. *Best Practice and Research: Clinical Gastroenterology* 18: 525–539.

9. Gevers et al. 2014 The treatment-naïve microbiome in new-onset Crohn's disease. *Cell Host and Microbe* 3: 383–392 is an excellent recent work examining the influence of community balance on IBD. A less technical summary of the research can be found at www.sciencedaily.com/releases/2014/03/140312132617.htm.

10. The role of peacemaker bacteria as well as their depletion in sufferers of Crohn's disease can be read in Velasquez-Manoff 2015 Gut

Microbiome: The Peacekeepers. *Nature* 518: S3–S11 and can also be seen diagrammatically in Your microbes at work: fiber fermenters keep us healthy in *Nature* 518: S9.

11. This community alteration is discussed in the references in note 9 above.

12. The complex role of antibiotics in helping and hindering Crohn's disease and its complications is discussed by Bernstein 2013 Antibiotic use and the risk of Crohn's disease. *Gastroenterology and Hepatology* 9: 393–395. The role of antibiotics in IBD generally has been the subject of much debate that largely stems from the fact that they can be very useful in some cases and less so in others.

13. A role for the gut microbiota in IBS is considered in a review paper of the same title by Collins 2014 *Nature Reviews Gastroenterology & Hepatology* 11: 497–505.

14. IBS and enhanced pain perception was studied by Tillisch and Mayer 2005 Pain perception in irritable bowel syndrome. *CNS Spectrums* 10: 877–882. A fascinating array of psychoemotional complications of IBS, including a fear of failure, the ready acceptance of a subordinate position and tension can be found in Dragos et al. 2012 Psychoemotional features in irritable bowel syndrome. *Journal of Medicine and Life* 15: 398–409.

15. Discussed in Collins 2014 (see note 13 above).

16. Germfree animals are raised in isolation from the external environment and are entirely free of colonising bacteria, both inside and out. We met germfree mice in Chapter Six.

17. This surprising result, which should be taken into account when considering faecal microbiota transplants such as those discussed in Chapter Ten, is published in Collins et al. 2013 The adoptive transfer of behavioral phenotype via the intestinal microbiota: experimental evidence and clinical implications. *Current Opinion in Microbiology* 16: 240–245.

Chapter 8: It's not my diet, doctor, it's my bacteria

1. You can access Fact sheet No. 311 through the World Health Organization at www.who.int/mediacentre/factsheets/fs311/en/.

2. This fascinating research can be read in Goodrich et al. 2014 Human genetics shape the gut microbiome. *Cell* 789–799. The research was widely covered in the media and the press release from Cornell, *Gut bacteria: how genes determine the fit of your jeans*, can be read at mediarelations.cornell.edu/2014/11/06/gut-bacteria-how-genes-determine-the-fit-of-your-jeans/.

3. The surprising fact that identical twins can differ genetically is highlighted by research by Li et al 2014 Somatic point mutations occurring early in development: a monozygotic twin study. *Journal of Medical Genetics* 51: 28–34. A popular account of this research can be found at www.livescience.com/24694-identical-twins-not-identical. html. Other research has revealed genetic differences between identical twins, some of which is covered in a highly readable article in *Scientific American* at www.scientificamerican.com/article/identical-twins-genes-are-not-identical/.

4. Although our gut microbiota can and does change over time and with factors like disease, its relative stability over time and in the face of lifestyle and diet changes is revealed by many studies including: Martinez et al. 2013 Long-term temporal analysis of the human fecal microbiota revealed a stable core of dominant bacterial species. *PLoS ONE* DOI: 10.1371/journal.pone.0069621. Some researchers really got their hands dirty with a daily follow-up of subjects' poo: Durbán et al. 2012 Daily follow-up of bacterial communities in the human gut reveals stable composition and host-specific patterns of interaction. *FEMS Microbiology Ecology* 81: 427–437. The stability of the gut community is also discussed by Lozupone et al. 2012 Diversity, stability and resilience of the human gut microbiota. *Nature* 489: 220–230, which also highlights the important fact that 'Viewing the microbiota from an ecological perspective could provide insight

into how to promote health by targeting this microbial community in clinical treatments'.

5. These findings are published in Goodrich et al. 2014 Human genetics shape the gut microbiome. *Cell* 789–799.

6. Mice microbiota is again the model system, this time in research by Carmody et al. 2015 Murine gut microbiota – diet trumps genes. *Cell Host and Microbe* 17: 72–84.

7. The role of brown fat and gut bacteria can be read in Mestdagh et al. 2012 Gut microbiota modulate the metabolism of brown adipose tissue in mice. *Journal of Proteome Research* 11: 620-630 and a more accessible account can be found at www.medicalnewstoday.com/articles/241725.php.

8. The benefit of eating apples for preventing heart attacks and stroke was studied by Briggs and Mizdrak 2013 A statin a day keeps the doctor away: comparative proverb assessment modelling study. *British Medical Journal* 18 December 2013. It is also covered in *An apple a day keeps vascular mortality at bay, study suggests* at www.medicalnewstoday.com/articles/270298.php.

9. Butyric acid-producing anaerobic bacteria as a novel probiotic treatment approach for inflammatory bowel disease is covered in a paper with this title by Van Immerseel et al. 2010 in the *Journal of Medical Microbiology* 59: 141–143.

10. The prebiotic value of different apples can be read in Condezo-Hoyos et al. 2014 Assessing non-digestible compounds in apple cultivars and their potential as modulators of obese faecal microbiota in vitro. *Food Chemistry* 161: 208–215. It is also discussed in *Could an apple a day protect against obesity* at www.medicalnewstoday.com/articles/283223.php.

11. This absolutely fascinating research was by Chen et al. 2014 Incorporation of therapeutically modified bacteria into gut microbiota inhibits obesity. *The Journal of Clinical Investigation* 124: 3391–3406. A summary and some insight from the research team can be found at news.vanderbilt.edu/2014/07/bacteria-prevent-obesity/.

12. These sage words are quoted in *Could a probiotic prevent obesity* at www.medicalnewstoday.com/articles/280078.php.

Chapter 9: Why it's good to stay in touch with 'old friends'

1. The global increase in asthma is highlighted in the World Health Organization's Factsheet No. 206 available at www.who.int/mediacentre/factsheets/fs206/en/.

2. The paper by David Strachan is Strachan 1989 Hay fever, hygiene and household size. *British Medical Journal* 299: 1259–1260.

3. This point is covered in the excellent review *The Hygiene Hypothesis and its implications for home hygiene, lifestyle and public health*, written by Rosalind Smith, Sally Bloomfield and Graham Rook (watch out for his name in association with the 'Old Friends' hypothesis) and published by the International Forum of Home Hygiene in 2012. This is well worth a read if the topic interests you. It's comprehensive and technical in places, but overall very approachable, readable and informative.

4. Some of the relationships between family size and allergic diseases are discussed by the originator of the idea, David Strachan, in Strachan 2000 Family size, infection and atopy: the first decade of the 'hygiene hypothesis'. *Thorax* 55: Supplement 1 S2–S10. He sums up the relationship by saying that the 'inverse association of family size with allergic sensitisation remains an enigmatic but potentially informative lead in the search for underlying causes of the rising prevalence of atopic disease in Western societies'. You can also read some discussion of this point in the reference in notes 3 and 5 to this chapter.

5. Another good read if you are interested in this topic, this reference is Bloomfield et al. 2006 Too clean or not too clean: the Hygiene Hypothesis and home hygiene. *Clinical and Experimental Allergy* 36: 402–425.

6. This review is *The Hygiene Hypothesis and its implications for home hygiene, lifestyle and public health* by Rosalind Smith, Sally Bloomfield

and Graham Rook published by the International Forum of Home Hygiene in 2012 (also footnote 3 this chapter).

7. Smith et al. 2012, mentioned in note 3, suggest that social changes in the late twentieth century have led to a more superficial approach to home cleaning, where speed, ease and appearing to be clean are more important than preventing disease.

8. Discussed in Bloomfield et al. 2006 Too clean or not too clean: the Hygiene Hypothesis and home hygiene (see note 5 above).

9. This fascinating research can be read in Kondrashova et al. 2005 A six-fold gradient in the incidence of type 1 diabetes at the eastern border of Finland. *Annals of Medicine* 37: 67–72.

10. The 'Old Friends' hypothesis is first put forward in Rook et al 2004 Mycobacteria and other environmental organisms as immunomodulators for immunoregulatory disorders. *Springer Seminars in Immunopathology* 25: 237–255.

11. Graham Rook provides an excellent overview of the 'Old Friends' hypothesis in 'A Darwinian view of the hygiene or 'Old Friends' hypothesis', published in 2012 in the journal *Microbe* 7: 173–180.

12. This notion is discussed by Graham Rook in the reference cited in note 10, and in references mentioned within that paper.

13. Anti-inflammatory treatment for depression is examined in a meta-review (which analyses data from many different studies) by Köhler et al. 2014 Effect of anti-inflammatory treatment on depression, depressive symptoms, and adverse effects: A systematic review and meta-analysis of randomized clinical trials. *JAMA Psychiatry* 71: 1381–1391. Cytokines and depression are discussed in light of the 'Old Friends' hypothesis by Rook in the reference in note 10.

14. Research linking autism and gut bacteria, and other connections between our brain and our internal ecosystem, are discussed in Schmidt 2015 Mental health: Thinking from the gut. *Nature Innovations in the Microbiome* 518: S12–S15.

Chapter 10: Are you really going to eat that?

1. The news release from the FDA entitled 'United States enters consent decree prohibiting illegal distribution of Luvena Prebiotic products', issued 30 January 2015, can be read at www.fda.gov/NewsEvents/Newsroom/PressAnnouncements/ucm432505.htm.

2. Prebiotic as a concept was introduced in Gibson and Roberfroid 1995 Dietary modulation of the human colonic microbiota: introducing the concept of prebiotics. *The Journal of Nutrition* 125: 1401–1412.

3. Analysis of various fruits and vegetables as sources of prebiotics was undertaken by Jovanovic-Malinovska et al. 2014 Oligosaccharide profile in fruits and vegetables as sources of prebiotics and functional foods. *International Journal of Food Properties* 5: 949–965.

4. A further review of prebiotics in foods as well as some useful information on the different roles of the many substances regarded to be prebiotic can be found in Al-Sharaji et al. 2013 Prebiotics as functional foods: a review. *Journal of Functional Foods* 5: 1542–1553.

5. A very useful single source here is Gibson et al. 2010 Dietary prebiotics: current status and new definition. *Food Science and Technology Bulletin: Functional Foods* 7: 1–19.

6. Some insights into this area of research are provided by DiBaise et al. 2012 Impact of the gut microbiota on the development of obesity: current concepts. *The American Journal of Gastroenterology Supplements* 1: 22–27. Also, Da Silva et al. 2013 Intestinal microbiota; relevance to obesity and modulation by prebiotics and probiotics. *Nutrición Hospitalaria* 28: 1039–1048.

7. An excellent port of call for the latest developments in prebiotics is Rastall and Gibson 2015 Recent developments in prebiotics to selectively impact beneficial microbes and promote intestinal health. *Current Opinion in Biotechnology* 32: 42–46.

8. Insights into the fascinating scientific life of Ilya Ilyich Mechnikov

can be read at www.nobelprize.org/nobel_prizes/medicine/laureates/1908/mechnikov-bio.html

9. An interesting article on probiotics in general, with a UK-focus, can be read at www.theguardian.com/theguardian/2009/jul/25/probiotic-health-benefits.

10. The probiotics global market was valued at $26 billion in 2012 by Markets and Markets www.marketsandmarkets.com/PressReleases/probiotics.asp. Growth estimates can be found at www.marketsandmarkets.com/Market-Reports/probiotic-market-advanced-technologies-and-global-market-69.html.

11. A readable account of the European ban and its implications for the industry can be read at www.foodmanufacture.co.uk/Regulation/Probiotics-ban-leads-to-marketing-revolution. Some within the industry hold out hope that the ban might be reversed: see http://www.foodmanufacture.co.uk/Regulation/Probiotic-generic-descriptor-application-moves-on. A useful Q and A approach outlining the European situation is available at www.fsai.ie/faqs/probiotic_health_claims.html#approved_prebiotic_claim. Information on the FDA ban, as well as some interesting discussion of how regulation might limit research, can be read at www.sciencedaily.com/releases/2013/10/131017144630.htm.

12. The upper limit of insects in various commodities allowable in the US is given in the *Defect Levels Handbook* published by the FDA and accessible at www.fda.gov/food/guidanceregulation/guidancedocumentsregulatoryinformation/sanitationtransportation/ucm056174.htm. It's a genuinely engaging read. In ground pepper, for example, the Action Level is an 'Average of 475 or more insect fragments per 50 grams' and an 'Average of 2 or more rodent hairs per 50 grams'. Yummy!

13. An excellent summary of research into AAD and probiotics can be read at http://www.cochrane.org/CD004827/IBD_probiotics-for-the-prevention-of-pediatric-antibiotic-associated-diarrhea-aad.

14. The usefulness of probiotics in long-term *C. difficile* infections is discussed at http://www.cochrane.org/CD006095/IBD_the-

use-of-probiotics-to-prevent-c.-difficile-diarrhea-associated-with-antibiotic-use.

15. The benefit of 'Probiotics for prevention of necrotizing enterocolitis in preterm infants' can be read at http://www.cochrane.org/CD005496/NEONATAL_probiotics-for-prevention-of-necrotizing-enterocolitis-in-preterm-infants.

16. A review of probiotics and IBS was conducted by Moayyedi et al 2010 The efficacy of probiotics in the treatment of irritable bowel syndrome: a systematic review. *Gut* 59: 325–332. It concludes that 'Probiotics appear to be efficacious in IBS, but the magnitude of benefit and the most effective species and strain are uncertain'.

17. Information on probiotics in relation to lactose intolerance can be found at www.nhs.uk/Conditions/probiotics/Pages/Introduction.aspx#lactose.

18. For an extremely readable and balanced overview of probiotics as therapy in a range of conditions visit www.nhs.uk/Conditions/probiotics/Pages/Introduction.aspx.

19. FMT procedure, in this case for those with recurrent *C. difficile* infections, is given at www.nice.org.uk/guidance/ipg485/chapter/3-the-procedure. It is short and sweet, so worth quoting in full: 'Before the procedure, donors (who can be family members or unrelated) are screened for enteric bacterial pathogens, viruses and parasites. Donor faeces are taken and diluted with water, saline or another liquid such as milk or yogurt, and subsequently strained to remove large particles. The resulting suspension is introduced into the recipient's gut via a nasogastric tube, nasoduodenal tube, rectal enema or via the biopsy channel of a colonoscope. Recipients may receive a bowel lavage before transplantation, in order to reduce the *C. difficile* load in the intestines.'

20. Some of these opportunities are discussed in a very approachable review article by Smits et al 2013 Therapeutic potential of fecal microbiota transplantation. *Gastroenterology* 145: 946–953. They include 'irritable bowel syndrome, inflammatory bowel diseases, insulin resistance, multiple sclerosis, and idiopathic

thrombocytopenic purpura'. No, I'd not heard of it either – it's more commonly and more accurately called immune thrombocytopenia and it's an autoimmune disease involving blood platelets; people with it are more prone to bruising and bleeding. The authors also note that 'There has been increasing focus on the interaction between the intestinal microbiome, obesity, and cardiometabolic diseases, and ... We might someday be able to mine for intestinal bacterial strains that can be used in the diagnosis or treatment of these diseases.'

21. The astonishing success of FMT in treating C. *diff* infection is discussed by Bakken et al. 2011 Treating *Clostridium difficile* infection with fecal microbiota transplantation. *Clinical Gastroenterology and Hepatology* 9: 1044–1049.

22. The brave new world of FMT therapy is discussed in Borody and Khoruts 2012 Fecal microbiota transplantation and emerging applications. *Nature Reviews Gastroenterology and Hepatology* 9: 88–96.

23. Potential applications of FMT are detailed in Borody and Khoruts 2012 Fecal microbiota transplantation and emerging applications. *Nature Reviews Gastroenterology and Hepatology* 9: 88–96.

24. This remarkable study was undertaken by Smith et al 2013 Gut microbiomes of Malawian twin pairs discordant for kwashiorkor. *Science* 339: 548–554. An interesting article and something of a call to arms that features this research is Knight 2015 Why Microbiome Treatments Could Pay Off Soon. *Nature* 518: S5.

Glossary

Amino acid: the building blocks of proteins. They are made up of carbon, hydrogen, oxygen and, crucially, nitrogen atoms that are arranged in a configuration common to all amino acids. There are about 20 different amino acids in our bodies and these differ from each other by having different atoms in the so-called 'side group'. Chaining amino acids together in different combinations leads to a staggering variety of different proteins.

Antibiotic: any of a large number of different substances produced by bacteria and fungi that can kill or inhibit the growth of bacteria and other microorganisms. They are used medically to treat infectious diseases and include well-known medicines like penicillin and streptomycin.

Artefact: an observation or measurement that has arisen as a consequence of something 'unnatural' acting on the system in question. For example, an increase in a patient's blood pressure might be an artefact of the stress caused by having blood pressure measured rather than a consequence of any medical condition.

Asymptomatic colonisation: to be colonised by a given species of bacteria (or other microorganism) without showing the disease symptoms characteristic of that species; aka 'silent carriage'.

B-cells: also called B-lymphocytes, B-cells are a type of white blood cell, some of which produce antibodies to fight off infections cf. T-cells.

Bacteroides: a genus (a closely related group) of bacteria that comprise a substantial proportion of the gut bacterial community.

Bacteriophage: a virus that infects bacteria and replicates inside bacterial cells. They are important in the transfer of genetic material between bacteria in nature and this property also makes them very useful for genetic research.

Bacterium: very small, very numerous single-celled organisms lacking a nucleus. The plural is bacteria. cf prokaryote.

Campylobacter: a group of bacteria that are a common cause of food poisoning and a major concern if you eat raw chicken.

CDC: abbreviation for the United States Centers for Disease Control and Prevention, whose main aim is to protect public health and safety through the control and prevention of disease, injury and disability.

Clostridium: a group of bacteria including *Clostridium botulinum* that produces botulinum toxin, used in Botox injects but which can also cause botulism, a potentially fatal disease. *Clostrodium difficile* can thrive in the gut if other bacteria have been killed by antibiotics. Infection with *C. difficile* it is a major problem in healthcare facilities.

Commensalism: a relationship between two organisms where

one organism benefits from the other without affecting it cf. mutualism.

Community: in ecology, a community is a group of interacting (or potentially interacting) species living in the same place.

Coprophagy: eating faeces; from the Greek for 'eating faeces'. A person who engages in this activity is a coprophage.

Coprophilia: an abnormal, often sexual, interest in faeces; from the Greek for 'fondness for faeces'.

Correlation/causal relationship: two or more things are said to be correlated if they vary together. For example, height and weight correlate; taller people tend to weigh more than shorter people. This is a positive correlation but if taller people tended to weigh less than taller people it would be a negative correlation. Things can be correlated without there being any *causal relationship* between them, in other words, one thing does not cause the other. This leads to the statistical adage that 'correlation does not imply causation'. For example, there is a very convincing correlation between the amount of margarine consumed and the divorce rate in the US state of Maine (widely reported, e.g. www.bbc.co.uk/news/magazine-27537142) but there is no sensible causal relationship between these things.

Cross-infection/cross-contamination: the unintended transfer of harmful microorganisms between people, especially within a healthcare setting, is cross-infection. Cross-contamination is the unintentional transfer of harmful microorganisms from one substance, object or surface to another.

Cytoplasm: the jelly-like material that makes up much of the inside of a cell.

E. coli: the bacterium Escherichia coli, common in the lower intestine of mammals and birds. Most strains are harmless although some can cause serious food poisoning and infections including urinary tract infections (UTIs).

Endospore: an exceptionally tough, stripped-down structure that is produced inside the cells of some bacterial species and can survive dormant for very long periods of time (in some cases centuries).

Enzyme: a protein produced by a cell, and coded for by a gene, that acts as a catalyst in a specific chemical reaction. Catalysts speed up reactions and without enzymes exerting their control over the biochemical processes within cells, life as we know it would not be possible. (Enzymes are also found in biological washing powders, where they assist in the breakdown of stains that have a biological origin.)

Epithelial cells: these cells make up epithelial tissue, one of the four basic tissue types in animals (the others being muscle tissue, nervous tissue and connective tissue), epithelial tissues form membranous linings to structures and cavities in the body.

Eukaryote: an organism made from cells that have a nucleus, as well as a well-developed internal membrane system and structures collectively termed organelles. Large, complex cells, this is the cell type found in plants, animals and fungi cf. prokaryote.

Faecal–oral highway: poo-to-mouth transfer, typically from surfaces contaminated with poo and via our hands.

FDA: abbreviation for the United States Food and Drug Administration, a federal body that enforces laws and regulations relating to food, drugs and cosmetics.

Flora: generally the plants of a particular region, habitat or geological period but sometimes also used in the same way to describe microorganisms.

Gene expression: the processes by which the information contained in the genetic code of a gene is used by a cell to make a 'gene product', usually a protein.

Genome: an organism's complete set of DNA, including all of its genes.

Genotype: the genetic makeup or constitution of an organism cf. phenotype.

Incidence: a measure of the probability that a person will be diagnosed with a given medical condition within a specified time. Incidence gives us an idea of the risk of contracting the condition cf. prevalence

In-vironment: a term sometimes used to mean the 'internal environment', typically the environment within the gut.

Listeria: Listeria monocytogenes is a bacterium that can cause food poisoning and other disease through contaminated food.

Listeriosis is the name given to the infection it causes.

Lymphocyte: a small white blood cell (leukocyte) important in the development of immunity. B-cells and T-cells are two specific types of lymphocyte cf. neutrophil.

Microbiome: the collective microorganisms and, crucially, their genetic material present in or on an environment. Typically it refers to the microorganisms (especially bacteria) present within the human body, or a part of the human body, e.g. 'gut microbiome' cf. microbiota.

Microbiota: the microorganisms present in a particular location, e.g. the human gut microbiota cf. microbiome.

Microflora: less commonly used alternative for microbiota that formally also includes microscopic algae.

Mitochondria: a bacterium-sized structure, or organelle, found in varying numbers within eukaryotic cells. The biochemistry of respiration takes place within them and for this reason they are sometimes called the 'power houses' of cells. As well as being bacterial in size and shape, they contain DNA and a genome that is similar to some bacterial genomes. According to the endosymbiont theory (the currently best-supported theory accounting for the existence of mitochondria) they are the remnants of bacteria taken in by ancient cells as food but which ended up working in a mutualistic partnership.

MRSA: methicillin-resistant *Staphylococcus aureus*, a strain of bacterium that causes potentially life-threatening infections but which is resistant to a number of widely used antibiotics. An example of a 'superbug', MRSA infections are more common in people in healthcare settings.

Mutualism: an ecological relationship between organisms of different species that is beneficial to those organisms cf. commensalism.

Mycobacteria: bacteria of the genus *Mycobacterium* that includes the bacteria responsible for tuberculosis and leprosy.

Neutrophil: a very common type of white blood cell that is one of the first responders to an infection site, where they attack invading microorganisms.

NHS: abbreviation for the UK's National Health Service, a publicly funded universal healthcare system.

Nosocomial infections: an infection originating in a hospital or other healthcare setting.

Pathogenic: an organism is pathogenic if it can, or does, cause disease. Pathogenicity is the ability of an organism to cause disease.

Phage: commonly used abbreviation for bacteriophage.

Phagocyte: a type of cell capable of engulfing and absorbing waste, foreign bodies and invading bacteria in the bloodstream and tissues.

Pilus: a hair-like appendage (plural, pili) found on the surface of many bacteria and used for attaching to surfaces (Type IV pili) or for transferring DNA between bacteria during conjugation (conjugative or conjugation pili).

Plasmid: a circular piece of DNA found in a bacterium separate from the DNA in the bacterial chromosome. Plasmids can be transferred between bacteria and are often the site for genes that confer resistance to antibiotics.

Prebiotic: any substance that promotes the existence and growth of beneficial microorganisms, most commonly used in reference to bacteria in the gut cf. probiotic.

Prevalence: the proportion of a population that has a disease at any given time. Prevalence gives us an idea of how widespread the condition is cf. incidence.

Probiotic: a preparation that contains bacteria designed to restore beneficial bacteria to the gut cf. prebiotic.

Prokaryote: a single-celled organism that lacks a nucleus, mitochondria or any other membrane-bound structures (organelles). Bacteria are prokaryotic cells cf. eukaryote.

Prophylactic dosing: an infection originating in a hospital or other healthcare setting.

Salmonella: a genus of bacteria in the same family as *E. coli* that is found in cold-blooded and warm-blooded animals, some strains of which cause food poisoning and typhoid fever.

Selenomonads: a group of bacteria commonly found in the guts of animals, especially ruminants like cattle and sheep.

Shiga toxin: a toxin produced by the bacterium *Shigella dysenteriae* that causes dysentery. A similar toxin, called Shiga-like toxin, is produced by some strains of *E. coli*.

Species: a group of organisms consisting of similar individuals capable of interbreeding to produce viable, fertile offspring.

Staphylococcus: a genus of bacteria that includes many pathogenic strains that cause the formation of pus, especially in the skin. Most of the time infection by these bacteria causes no problems or results in only minor skin infections but an infection that invades more deeply into the bloodstream, joints, bones, lungs or heart can be life threatening. MRSA is a strain of a species of *Staphylococcus aureus*.

Streptococcus te: a species of bacteria common in the human mouth and the major cause of tooth decay.

T-cells: also called T-lymphocytes, T-cells are a type of white blood cell crucial for the adaptive immune system that tailors the body's immune system to specific threats. T-cells are sometimes likened to soldiers, seeking out and destroying invading microorganisms cf. B-cells.

Teixobactin: a recently discovered small molecule that acts as an antibiotic against some bacteria. It was discovered using a new method of culturing bacteria in soil.

Tra: short for 'transfer gene', tra genes are necessary for the transfer of genetic material between bacteria.

Transduction: the transfer of viral DNA, bacterial DNA or both from one cell to another especially via a bacteriophage.

Treg cells: or Tregs, short for regulatory T cells. They regulate the immune system by supressing the function of other T-cells, thereby preventing excessive reactions.

Triclosan: an antibacterial and antifungal agent widely found in products such as soap, toys, mouthwashes, kitchen utensils and toys whose use is regulated in many territories, primarily because of concerns about bacterial resistance. It is also debateable whether it is much more effective than soap and water in many applications.

WHO: abbreviation for World Health Organization, the public health arm of the United Nations that monitors disease outbreaks, assesses heath system performance and promotes health worldwide.

Zoonosis: a disease that can be transmitted from animals to people.

Index